KU-496-921

Clinical Techniques in Dentistry

An Atlas of
Minor Oral Surgery

Principles and Practice

DISPOSED OF FROM
CWM TAF LIBRARY
SERVICES 2024
NEWER INFORMATION
MAYBE AVAILABLE

Books are to be returned on or before
the last date below.

17 APR 2001

14 JAN 2002

25 MAR 2008

LIBREX—

E00181

Clinical Techniques in Dentistry

An Atlas of Minor Oral Surgery

Principles and Practice

David A McGowan

MDS, PhD, FDSRCS, FFDRCSI, FDSRCPSG

Professor of Oral Surgery
University of Glasgow

MARTIN DUNITZ

© David A McGowan 1989

First published in 1989 by
Martin Dunitz Ltd, The Livery House, 7-9 Pratt Street, London NW1 0AE
Reprinted 1991

All rights reserved. No part of this publication may be reproduced, stored in a retrieval system or transmitted in any form or by any means, without the prior permission of the publisher.

British Library Cataloguing in Publication Data

McGowan, David A., *1939–*
    An atlas of minor oral surgery.
    I. Man. Oral region. Surgery
    I. Title
    617.'522059
    ISBN 0–948269–65–0

EAST GLAMORGAN GENERAL HOSPITAL
CHURCH VILLAGE. near PONTYPRIDD

Laserset by Scribe Design, Gillingham, Kent
Originated, printed and bound by Toppan Printing Company (S) Pte Ltd, Singapore

Contents

Preface

Despite the success of prevention, and the improvement in dental health in many parts of the world, the ability to extract teeth is still a necessary skill for most dentists. Patients do not relish the experience, but control of anxiety, avoidance of pain and reduction of discomfort will earn their gratitude. As in any form of surgery, complications must arise from time to time, and the dentist who undertakes to extract teeth has to be prepared to meet them. The skills, equipment and practice organization required for these purposes can be usefully employed in preplanned dento-alveolar surgery, and this continuing activity in turn ensures efficiency of response when the need arises.

The purpose of this book is to promote a systematic and organized approach to minor oral surgery, while still allowing for variation in technique to suit personal preference, local circumstances and, most important of all, the needs of the individual patient. General principles are emphasized and illustrated by examples of the commoner procedures. 'Minor oral surgery' comprises those surgical operations which can comfortably be completed by a practised nonspecialist dentist in not more than 30 minutes under local anaesthesia. This defines the scope of the book. It is intended as a guide to all those who wish to learn, or improve their knowledge of this branch of the surgeon's art, but cannot replace the one-to-one instruction and guidance which the beginner requires. I hope to pass on some of the lessons learnt as a teacher of students and practitioners over a number of years and, in doing so, I dedicate this book to the patients in our dental schools and hospitals in recognition of their contribution to the advance of our profession.

Acknowledgments

I am indebted to many people for help with this book; to John Davies and the staff of the Department of Dental Illustration of Glasgow Dental Hospital and School, whose superb skills made the project possible; to my secretary, Sara Glen-Esk, who deciphered my scrawls and came to terms with the word-processor; to my consultant and junior colleagues, not only for helping me find and follow up suitable patients, but for the back-up which allowed me to find some time for writing; to the nursing staff who cared for the patients; to Harub Al-Kharusi and Ahmed Zahrani, who assisted with most of the cases; to Helen Shanks for duplicating the radiographs; to Gordon MacDonald and Jim Rennie for the pathology reports; and to my wife and family for their forbearance.

It has been a pleasure to work with the Martin Dunitz organization—and especially with Mary Banks.

I am also grateful to Bernard Smith, who first suggested that I might undertake this task.

DAMcG

Part 1   Principles

1 Diagnosis and treatment planning

All surgery produces tissue damage and patient morbidity, so every operation must be justified by weighing benefit against detriment. There is no such thing as a 'routine' operation. The purpose must be one of the following:

- elimination of disease
- prevention of future disease or disadvantage
- removal of damaged or redundant tissue
- improvement of function or aesthetics.

To take a common example, the removal of a completely buried asymptomatic unerupted tooth or retained root fragment inflicts certain surgical damage and is not justified by the hypothetical risk of future infection. However, when there is a defect in the overlying mucosa, the balance of probability is completely altered and removal is advised.

Effective clinical decision-making depends on the gathering and objective analysis of relevant information, and then on judgment based on experience, instinct and, it must be admitted, even prejudice. The clinician can never allow him- or herself the certainty which patients demand.

A minor oral surgical operation is only one item in a patient's continuing dental care. The extraction of an impacted third molar, followed later by the extraction of the carious second molar which produced the symptoms in the first place, is not only foolish but damaging to the interests of both patient and dentist.

While diagnosis is a theoretical exercise, treatment planning must be responsive to the practical day-to-day realities of economic and social factors, and successful patient management depends on achieving the right balance.

Apart from the few purely soft tissue procedures, minor oral surgery diagnosis depends heavily on radiographs which are too often of poor quality and examined hastily. Acceptance of a low standard of radiographic diagnosis is frankly negligent.

Pre-operative assessment of difficulty cannot be exact, and the margin of error must always lie on the safe side. Overestimation of difficulty leads to relief and gratitude, while underestimation leads to embarrassment at least, and distress and litigation at worst. The general dentist who refers a difficult case to a specialist will earn the respect of both patient and colleague. With experience, the accuracy of assessment will increase and can be tailored to the increasing surgical competence of the operation.

Fitness for minor oral surgery

The dangers of minor oral surgery have been grossly exaggerated. Unnecessary apprehension has been aroused by a combination of dominant physicians ignorant of dentistry, and timid dentists ignorant of medicine. In fact, most of the fears experienced have little foundation. Excluding general anaesthesia, minor oral surgery under local anaesthesia, with or without sedation, is a remarkably safe undertaking.

It was formerly considered sufficient to believe that if a patient was fit enough to come to the surgery, they were fit enough to receive treatment – and the cautious sited their premises at the top of a flight of stairs! However, the success of modern medicine in keeping alive and active many patients who would have been at least bed-ridden in the past, has negated such a simple approach. From student days onwards, considerable efforts are made to educate dentists to a high level of knowledge and understanding of medicine, and it is now considered negligent to fail to obtain a current medical history and to appreciate its significance.

In case of concern, it is prudent to discuss potential problems with the patient's physician. It must, however, be remembered that advice once sought must be taken, and will always tend to err on the side of caution. Minor oral surgery, as defined in the preface to this book, does not include the treatment of patients who are obviously acutely ill, or the chronically sick, unless they are ambulant and able to live a relatively normal life. Chronic disease, which is well-controlled and stable, is unlikely to raise problems, but the often complex medication itself can raise the possibility of unfavourable drug interactions. However, 2 to 4 ml of one of the commonly-used local anaesthetic solutions containing 2 per cent lignocaine with 1/80 000 adrenaline (US: 2 per cent lidocaine with 1/80 000 epinephrine) will not be harmful.

It is far more important to treat the patient with kindness and consideration, and to avoid the stress which triggers the release of endogenous catecholamines, than to complicate the issue by using allegedly safer preparations of less certain efficacy.

For a detailed discussion of the subject, the reader is referred to one of the many textbooks available which discuss the myriad possibilities at great length. Some recommended texts are listed in the Recommended Reading section.

2 Pre-operative preparation

Thorough preparation is the key to successful surgery, and the various aspects to be considered will be discussed in turn (see table below), but all the links in the chain are interdependent. Efficiency wins, and maintains, patients' confidence and co-operation. Difficulties arise more often from lack of planning, or forethought, than from any lack of manual skill.

Pre-operative check list

Patient
- Comfortable – physically and mentally relaxed
- Anaesthetized ± sedated – verbal
  - oral
  - intravenous
  - inhalational
- Informed consent
- Information – case records
  - radiographs

Equipment
- Light
- Suction
- Instruments
- Dressing/medicaments

Assistant
- Trained/informed

Operator
- Pre-operative assessment
- Operation plan
- Contingency plans

The patient

No one looks forward with pleasure to surgery, however minor, and perhaps the best that can be hoped for is indifference. Patients will be apprehensive to a variable extent and deserve sympathetic reassurance. Most fears will be alleviated by discussion, but shyness or shame about showing fear may impede communication. A patient must consent, at least verbally, to undergo the planned treatment. This can be done properly only if he or she has received an explanation of the operation, its purpose and procedure, and of the consequences, including an assessment of possible harmful effects. Radiographs are a great aid to explanation, and should be shown to the patient. An appraisal of the degree of sedation required needs to be made in advance, and the social consequence of both the operation and sedation discussed. On the operation day, the patient should obviously be received in a courteous, unhurried manner and seated comfortably in the chair. If possible, he or she should be accompanied home afterwards by a responsible adult.

Case records should be checked and placed in a position where they can be readily consulted during the operation without the necessity for handling. Radiographs must be properly illuminated and checked for correct identity and orientation in every case.

The equipment

The instrument kit required will vary with the demands of the procedure and the operator's preference. A suitable surgical kit is listed and illustrated in Appendix A (page 126). Instruments should be prepared and sterilized in kits, and will remain sterile if stored dry in a closed pack.

Two fundamental requirements, which cannot be overemphasized, are effective lighting and suction – good surgery is impossible without both and, when difficulty is encountered, the automatic response should be to check vision and exposure before taking any other action. While lighting is equally important for other dental procedures, suction for surgical purposes should be of the high vacuum/low volume type to ensure the efficient removal of blood, as well as the saline irrigation. A large bore, high-volume apparatus produces drying of the wound and also carries the risk of the loss of small fragments of tooth or soft tissue, which should be retained for examination. Cutting equipment should be tested before the patient is brought in, and any dressings or medicaments required be made ready in advance.

The assistant

Minor oral surgery is a 'four-handed' procedure, and skilled assistance is vital. Most dental assistants enjoy the variety and the challenge of this kind of work, but need special training to be able to cope with the extra demands of the often apprehensive patient and the necessity for rigorous sterility. It is obviously vital to explain the operation plan to the assistant in advance.

The operator

The operator needs to be clear as to how he or she intends to proceed. Most, though not all, problems can be anticipated. The information obtained from the original history and examination, supplemented by radiography, is the basis of the operation plan required for a preliminary explanation to the patient and assistant. As the operation proceeds — particularly as the tissues are dissected and retracted — the options become clearer and a change of plan may be needed.

The patient should be positioned so as to give the operator a clear view and a comfortable working position.

3   The operation

All minor oral surgery operations follow a similar sequence of stages, which is the basis of a systematic approach (see table below). Adherence to a logical overall plan is a great help when difficulties arise. Like any other surgery, the sequence follows the anatomical tissue planes — first inwards until the objective is achieved, and then outward until the wound is repaired.

Stages of the operation sequence

- Retraction
- Incision
- Reflection
- Bone removal – access
            – point of elevation
            – removal of obstruction
- Tooth section
- Delivery
- Clean-up
- Sew-up
- Check-up
- Follow-up
- Write-up

Retraction

The first procedure is the placement of a suitable retractor so as to display the operation site and hold the lips, cheeks and tongue out of the way. The Kilner cheek retractor will control both lips and cheek, provided it is held at the correct angle so as to pouch out the cheek. The tongue is best controlled by ignoring it — conscious efforts by the patient are seldom helpful. When the retractor is in place, a final check should be made on the relative positions of the patient, the operator, the assistant, and the light.

Incision

The shape of the incision has to be planned with the needs of both exposure and closure in mind. A long incision heals as easily as a short one, and so exposure should be generous. While the mental nerve is the only significant structure at risk, thoughtful placement of incisions can reduce haemorrhage by avoiding unnecessary section of muscles or small constant vessels. Most incisions can be made on to the underlying bone, and this ensures separation of both mucosal and periosteal layers in the one cut. The hand should be steadied, if possible, by using a suitable rest for the fingers. Incisions may sometimes be conveniently extended with tissue scissors.

Reflection

The mucoperiosteal flap is reflected with a periosteal elevator, such as a Howarth's. Two elevators can be used to advantage at this stage — one working and the other aiding retraction in the subperiosteal plane. Adequate undermining of the wound margins is required in order to mobilize the flap. Generous reflection is the key to adequate vision, and wide exposure reduces traction trauma to the wound edges.

Bone removal

Removal of bone is usually required and, in the interest of vision and to reduce trauma from excessive elevating force, should be generous. This is most conveniently achieved by using a bur in a slow- to moderate-speed handpiece. Handheld chisels are useful in 'peeling off' thin layers of bone, and rongeurs are ideal when the blades can be placed either side of the piece of bone to be removed. Bone files are seldom required since sharp edges can be 'nibbled' off. Excessive smoothing is unnecessarily traumatic and time-wasting.

Although generous in extent, bone removal must be calculated to achieve an end, and never be blindly destructive. The main objectives should be the achievement of access, the establishment of a point of application for an elevator (or forceps), and the removal of the obstruction to movement of the tooth or root. It may be that all these objectives may be reached simultaneously, but in any event they should be considered in that order. Slots or gutters around teeth or roots should be deep and narrow so as to preserve a fulcrum for leverage. Additionally the shape of the tooth must be borne in mind, both when clearing the cardinal points of the crown and in allowing for curvature and angulation of the roots.

Tooth section

Division of a tooth into a number of simpler, or more favourably shaped, segments may resolve the conflicts of the paths of withdrawal, or relieve impaction. This is best achieved by piercing the surface with a round bur, which is then sunk to the estimated width of the tooth, and the round 'shaft' converted into a slot with a fissure bur. Tungsten carbide tipped burs are essential for efficient cutting. The depth of all cuts should be judged so as to remain within tooth substance, and to avoid damage to the neighbouring structures. Final separation is achieved by levering within the slot with a flat elevator until the tooth cracks apart. In order to avoid propagating the crack through the bone, it is safer to gain even limited movement of the tooth within the socket before section.

Delivery

When all necessary bone removal and tooth section is complete, the tooth or root is delivered, usually by leverage with an elevator. When the root form is complicated, and there is marked curvature in more than one plane, withdrawal with forceps may be easier, provided that they can be applied. The successful delivery of the tooth is a cause of some satisfaction, and is usually greeted with relief by the patient, but this does not represent the end of the operation! The stages which follow are calculated to ensure trouble-free healing, and are just as important as those already completed.

Pathological specimens are welcomed by the oral pathology departments of most dental schools. They will provide suitable containers, advise on postal service rules on packing and despatch and report on specimens — usually without charge.

Clean-up

The socket, or other bony defect, should be examined for the presence of debris — pieces of enamel, amalgam, calculus or loose chips of bone all seem to delay healing until exfoliated. Soft tissue tags can be removed with discretion, although there is no evidence that they cause any harm. Excessive irrigation is unnecessary and washes away adherent clotted blood, which is the best dressing material available. Bleeding points may need to be clipped but, fortunately, significant haemorrhage is very rare and ligation, which is often extremely difficult, is seldom required. Persistent oozing will respond to packing with a swab, and to patience.

When bleeding is controlled, and the wound is clean, it is then ready for closure.

Sew-up

Most minor oral surgical wounds are sutured so as to replace the flap in the optimum position for healing. The object is not to pull the edges together to form a tight seal, but rather to support them in position and prevent displacement in the early phase of healing. Reducing the gape of the defect also serves to decrease the chance of ingress of food debris, and gentle traction on the tissues will hold them firmly to the bone surface and stop them bleeding. The fewer the number of sutures used to produce the desired result, the better. Insertion of too many sutures tears the tissue unnecessarily, and the resulting tangle of suture thread tends to accumulate plaque and promote inflammation. Suture ends should not be cut too short, but rather left tied in an accessible position for later removal.

Check-up

On completion of suturing, the tension of retraction should be released and the wound re-examined for any gaping. A short period of pressure, applied by biting gently on a damp swab, will ensure the final cessation of haemorrhage. During this time, the patient's postoperative instructions may be discussed. It is prudent to use a set of brief, printed instructions, since memory can be fallible under such circumstances, and a suggested format for an advice leaflet is listed in Appendix C. Patients must understand how to keep the wound clean, with frequent saline mouth baths, and know how to get help if they suffer haemorrhage, severe pain or excessive swelling. Proscription of mouth-cleaning or rinsing, or of taking fluids by mouth, or taking alcohol in moderation, or indeed of smoking is unkind and unnecessary as there is no evidence that any of these practices have the slightest effect on initial wound healing. Nevertheless, excess should (as always) be avoided. Suitable analgesics should be given, or prescribed, and sensible restriction of activity and rest at home overnight advised.

Follow-up

A return appointment must be made before the patient is discharged. Seven days is usually the most convenient interval, but postponement for a few extra days is of no consequence. Earlier review, except in response to problems, should be avoided as healing to the point of reasonable comfort usually needs this 7-day interval.

Write-up

Brief, but accurate, operation notes must be made to record the procedure used, and to note any variation from the usual technique. Involvement of significant vessels or nerves, an account of broken apices and the number of sutures inserted, are all particularly important. A dramatic description is unnecessary and it is best rather to concentrate on those factors most likely to be significant in the long-term follow-up. All such notes must, of course, be dated and clearly signed, since they constitute the legal as well as the clinical record of the operation.

4   Postoperative care

A wise oral surgeon once remarked, 'The operation is finished when the patient stops complaining.' For most patients, the follow-up is short and untroubled, but for a few the consequences can be lifelong.

At the time of suture removal, patients need, above all, to be assured that their progress is normal and that the residual discomfort, swelling or trismus are as expected. They should be encouraged to look forward to early improvement.

The appearance of the sutures is in itself a valuable indicator of the success of the patient's wound care. Accumulation of plaque and debris, with resultant inflammation, tells its own tale. By no means do all minor oral surgical wounds heal by first intention and, in most cases, there will be granulating areas and often small defects where food fragments can lodge. Swabbing with damp cotton wool and flushing with saline or chlorhexidine solution will clean up the area and leave it much fresher for the patient.

Premature removal of sutures is difficult due to swelling, and perhaps trismus, although it can be a relief to the patient if there is gross oedema and the sutures have been tied tightly. Convenient, and therefore comfortable, suture removal requires the same conditions as the original surgery – retraction, light, suitable instruments and skilled assistance. Many patients fear the procedure and they can really be reassured only by painless removal of the first suture. Scissors must be sharp right up to the points, and non-toothed tissue forceps are best for holding and withdrawing the cut threads. Even if sutures have not been inserted, it is essential that the progress of healing is reviewed at about one week post-operation, and the wound may benefit from irrigation or dressing. Large defects may be packed with iodoform ribbon gauze, which will stay fresh in the oral wound for some weeks. Smaller defects may benefit from regular flushing with a suitable syringe, and the patient may require instruction in this technique.

Most postoperative pain and swelling are due simply to surgical trauma and not infection, although bacterial contamination is inevitable at operation and thereafter. It is not logical to rely on antibiotics to compensate for surgical clumsiness, and they should only be prescribed in the following cases:

- where infection was present preoperatively
- where healing capacity is impaired
- where protection from bacteraemia is essential
- when surgical trauma is particularly severe.

Patients having teeth removed by surgical methods will not be immune from the occasional occurrence of a 'dry socket', but prescription of antibiotics should not be relied upon either to prevent or cure this distressing condition. Effective treatment requires irrigation, gentle packing with iodoform ribbon gauze and, most importantly, a generous prescription of potent analgesics. Nonsteroidal anti-inflammatory agents such as propoxyphen may have a specially effective role in such cases. If the pain persists, then packing with zinc-oxide/eugenol paste is justified as it does appear to relieve pain, albeit at the cost of prolonged wound healing and some local tissue necrosis.

Postoperative haemorrhage is unusual, especially if care is taken to ensure complete haemostasis before discharging the patient after the operation. In the unlikely event of a postoperative haemorrhage occurring, the surgeon must be available to give advice and help. In most cases, gentle pressure on the wound – achieved by biting on a damp cloth pack for 10–15 minutes – will compress the soft tissues on to the underlying bone and cope with the problem; sitting quietly and bed rest will also help. In more persistent or severe cases, the patient must return to the surgery for re-examination of the wound. It is important to reassure the patient, and their families, that the bleeding, while a nuisance, is not dangerous to their life or health.

When in the surgery, the requirements for effective treatment are the same as for the planned case, but they are more difficult to meet in the emergency situation, particularly outside normal working hours. The administration of local anaesthetic solution into the bleeding area is often dramatically effective in arresting the bleeding by vasoconstriction. It allows proper examination of the wound and further suturing, or packing, to proceed without pain. The theoretical danger of recurrence of bleeding after the vasoconstriction passes off is met by the local measures, which will continue to exert their effect. Sutures should be placed to compress tissue at sites where grasping with tissue forceps reduces bleeding. A modest increase in suture tension is justified when the purpose is haemostasis.

Persistent oozing may respond to packing with oxidized cellulose gauze. This material forms a matrix for promotion of blood clotting and has no mechanical effect. Very rarely, a vascular bleeding point may be identified and clipped with a haemostat. Direct ligation of small vessels is very difficult to achieve, and a light binding suture around the tissue containing the vessel will usually be more feasible, and hence more effective.

Restricted mouth-opening for one or two weeks after third molar removal is so common that all patients should be warned to expect it. Persistence of the problem is usually associated with slow healing and prolonged inflammation, and will resolve when the underlying inflammatory stimulus is removed. In some cases, trismus persists for months, although it is never permanent. Some of these cases are examples of the rare problems that arise after inferior dental block injections, due either to haemorrhage or infection of the needle track. There is no effective treatment, and much patience is therefore required of the sufferer, supported by the surgeon. Relief, when it comes, tends to be rapid, and this lends weight to the suggestion that the mechanism is reflex inhibition of movement provoked by a painful stimulus.

Alteration of sensation in the area supplied by the mental or lingual nerve can follow surgery in the mandible. Pre-operative radiography may give a prior warning of this danger, and the operation may be modified accordingly, or even avoided, if the indication for surgery is weak. Flaps raised in the region of the mental foramen should be reflected far enough to identify the position of the nerve, rather than risk damaging it while working blind. If, despite these precautions, damage does occur, then careful assessment of the postoperative symptoms is essential. The extent and degree of alteration in sensation must be carefully recorded so that recovery can be monitored accurately. Generally speaking, those cases where some recovery is apparent in a few days will probably return to normal in a few months, but when there is more delayed recovery – or indeed no improvement by the end of 9 to 12 months – then no further progress can be expected. It follows, therefore, that patients must consent to the operation knowing the possibility of altered sensation, which occurs in up to 5 per cent of cases of third molar removal. Fortunately, only one in ten of these cases suffer from permanently altered sensation.

Sympathetic and thoughtful postoperative care not only benefits the patient, but also enables the surgeon to appraise critically the results of his work. This personal audit is the duty of every ethical clinician.

Part 2   Practice

Introduction

The cases illustrated in the following chapters have been deliberately chosen, not as perfect examples, but rather to demonstrate one presentation of each type of problem and the application of the basic principles given in Part I to some real-life situations.

The problems chosen for illustration are those most likely to arise in a general dental practice, and that fall within the scope of the skills and limitations on time defined earlier. The general indications for each type of operation are not discussed specifi-cally, as they are either patently obvious or sufficiently exemplified in the cases chosen. A more extensive theoretical discussion is to be found in the texts listed in the Recommended Reading section.

Each patient is introduced by a case history and, where appropriate, a radiographic assessment. The operation photograph sequences have been chosen to tell the story with the minimum of accompanying text. The outcome of each procedure is also described and illustrated, where possible.

5 Retained roots

Retained upper lateral incisor root

RW, a 24-year-old computer programmer, was concerned about the appearance of his upper anterior teeth. He sought advice on the partially erupted upper right canine and the retained upper left lateral incisor root. The orthopantomograph, while imperfect, was sufficient to exclude any other pressing surgical problems, although an unerupted upper right third molar was present. In consultation with an orthodontist and a prosthodontist, it was agreed that this patient should be advised to have the lateral incisor root removed, the canine brought into full eruption by traction with a fixed orthodontic appliance, and bridges provided to replace the lateral incisors.

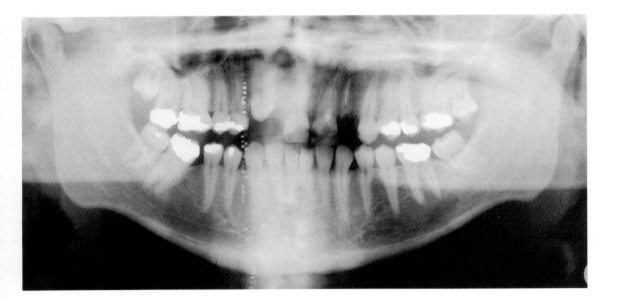

Radiographic assessment

The left upper lateral incisor root is small and conical, with substantial caries in the root face. The tooth has previously been root-filled and is likely to be brittle. There is some evidence of periapical disease. As removal looked to be otherwise easy, no further view was taken.

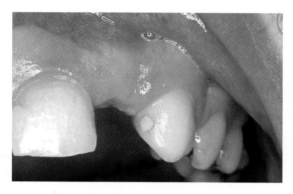

Operation

Operation site

There is a broad band of healthy attached gingivae with no defect.

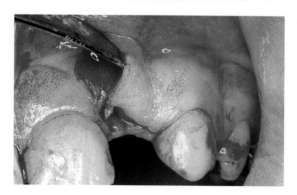

Incision

The papilla between the canine and the first premolar is released, and the incision carried round the gingival margin of the canine to the crest of the edentulous ridge mesially. It then runs along the crest to the distal of the central incisor. The relieving incision is made at a slightly obtuse angle and need only just cross the broad attached gingivae.

Reflection

The undermining of the flap commences at the relieving limb, using the curette end of a Mitchell's trimmer. This makes it easier to insert the broader, blunter Howarth's periosteal elevator, which is advanced along the bone and peels off the mucoperiosteal flap.

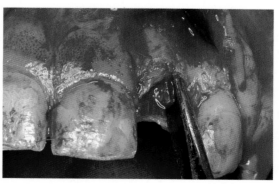

Elevation and delivery

The root can be clearly seen, and no overlying bone removal is necessary. A medium Coupland's chisel is used to loosen the root from its attachment mesially and distally, and to define the buccal and palatal margins prior to the application of forceps.

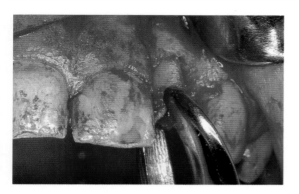

The root is easily removed, with care taken not to crush the hollow carious area between the blades.

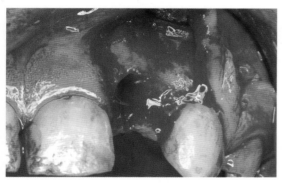

The socket

The socket is clean and the margins smooth.

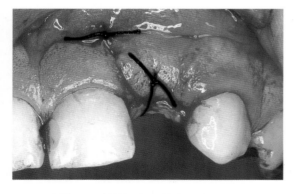

Closure

The first suture draws the flap into the mesial corner of the defect, and the second closes the gaping anterior relieving limb of the incision.

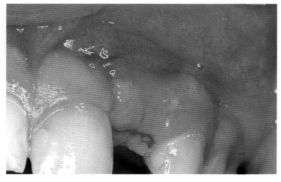

Follow-up

A week later, the sutures are removed and the area has healed well. There is some local plaque accumulation, and the patient needs to be encouraged to brush the area vigorously and not hold back for fear of damaging the healing wound.

Retained lower roots and unerupted third molar

YI, a 26-year-old female taxi driver, complained of infection of the sockets of the lower right molars which had been extracted some days before. There was marked inflammation in the area and gross aggregations of plaque and debris. The sockets were irrigated with chlorhexidine solution, hot saline mouthbaths advised, and a prescription for penicillin V given. One week later she was more comfortable, but considerable inflammation remained. Three months later she finally kept an appointment for the removal of the roots and the unerupted third molar.

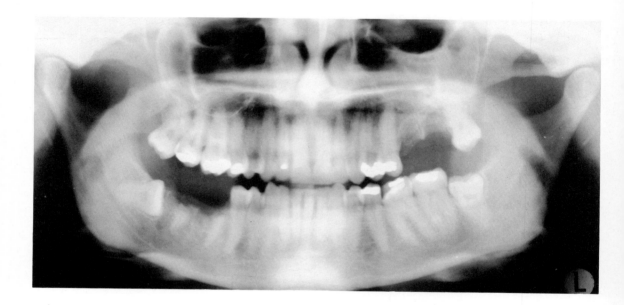

Radiographic assessment

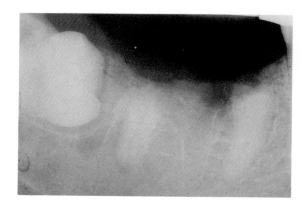

The retained fractured mesial roots of the lower right first and second molars can be clearly seen. Both are large, easy to find and simple in shape, and so easy to elevate. The third molar is in a horizontal position, with a tapering root shape, and its apex lies close to the inferior dental canal. Once the crown is uncovered, the tooth can be readily brought forward away from the canal and delivered into the space left by the extracted second molar roots, where bone removal will also release the mesial first molar root.

The orthopantomograph shows recurrent caries and destruction of other molars, and also a disto-angular lower left third molar. In view of the patient's poor cooperation, she was merely advised to have other treatment – more in hope than in expectation!

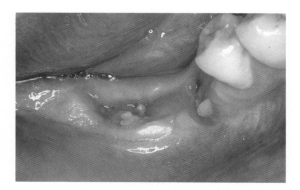

Operation

Operation site

Some minimal inflammation surrounds the jagged edges of the fractured first and second molar roots, but the third molar is completely covered. There is no keratinized buccal gingival tissue at the first molar root, and the flap will be friable in this area.

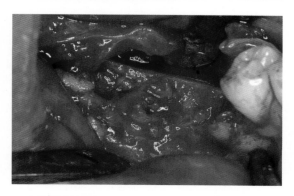

Incision

The incision runs forward from the thick fibrous tissue overlying the third molar, through the mucosal defects produced by the roots, to the distal gingival margin of the second premolar, and then down for a short way towards the sulcus to form an anterior corner.

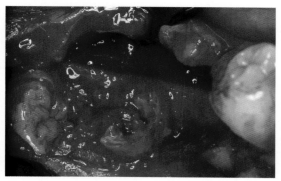

Reflection

The buccal and lingual tissues are reflected to give a clear view, and to enable the placement of a second Howarth's periosteal elevator as a lingual retractor. The roots are obscured by bleeding granulations which are curetted away.

Elevation and delivery of roots

The second molar root can now be clearly seen, and is easily elevated by mesial application of a Cryer's elevator, while the first molar root can be elevated backwards using a Coupland's chisel inserted mesially.

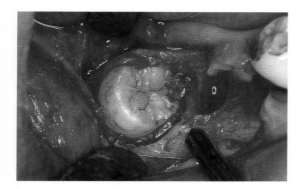

Bone removal

The roots and granulation tissue have been removed and the relationship of the third molar crown to the bone is now clearly visible. Some bone around the crown has been removed, using a small round bur in a 'guttering' technique.

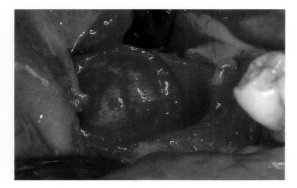

Elevation and delivery of third molar

The tooth is loosened and elevated out, using a Coupland's chisel.

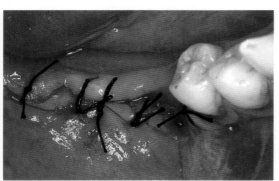

Socket

A clean socket is left.

Closure

The flap is replaced using five sutures. The first suture is placed to reposition the mesial corner, and the second is halfway along the incision. The other sutures approximate the gaping areas. As predicted, the flap cannot be completely closed in the first molar root region, and any further suturing here would merely tear the delicate buccal tissues.

Follow-up

The incision line healed satisfactorily and the patient was discharged following suture removal at one week.

Retained lower molar root

EL, a 45-year-old housewife, edentulous for 21 years, suffered intermittent pain in her left lower jaw for some months. When swelling developed, she sought help from her dental practitioner. He took a radiograph which raised the suspicion of a retained root in the third molar region. An antibiotic was prescribed, which resolved the acute problem, and she was referred for oral surgery. A small sinus opening in the mucosa could be seen and further radiographs showed the vague outline of a carious root. Exploration of the area was suggested, but declined by the patient. However, she reconsidered this decision a year later when the pain recurred, and then consented to have the root removed under local anaesthesia.

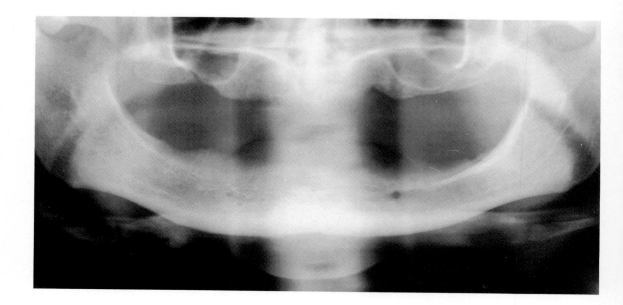

Radiographic assessment

The orthopantomograph shows the patient to be completely edentulous, and there is only a subtle indication of a root in the lower left third molar area. The periapical film is marginally more definite, and a straight outline can just be seen which represents the upper surface of the mesially-tilted root lying on the surface of the bone.

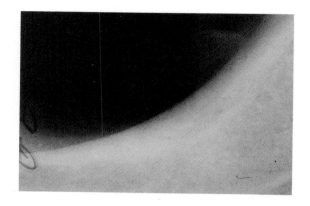

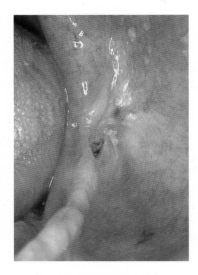

Operation

Operation site

A small mucosal defect lies just anterior to the retromolar pad, and the brown carious root surface can be seen within it. The flat edentulous mandible can be palpated beneath.

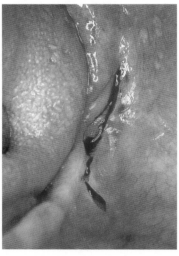

Incision

The incision commences posteriorly, just lateral to the retromolar pad, and runs through the defect along the buccal side of the crest of the ridge, to end in a deliberately angled short relieving branch.

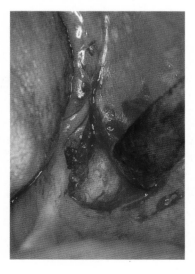

Reflection

The flap is reflected using a Howarth's elevator inserted first into the anterior relieving incision and then by stripping the soft tissues off the bone at the periosteal level.

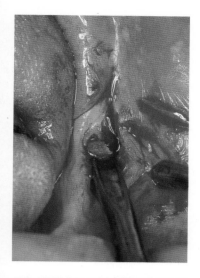

Elevation

The root can now be clearly seen, and is easily loosened with a Coupland's chisel.

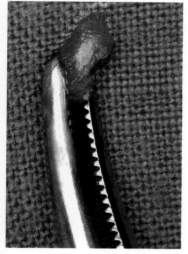

The root is lifted out with fine curved artery forceps.

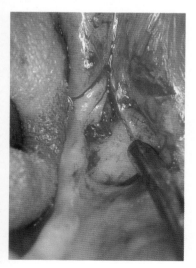

Socket

Residual scar and granulation tissue is curetted away with a Mitchell's trimmer.

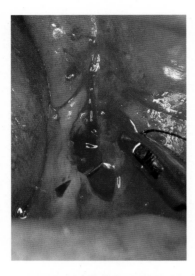

Closure

The incision is closed with two sutures, the first of which accurately repositions the flap in the original site by passing obliquely across the corner in the incision made for this purpose.

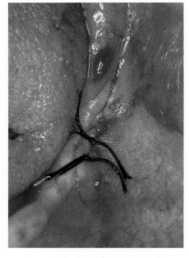

The second suture helps approximation and prevents gaping.

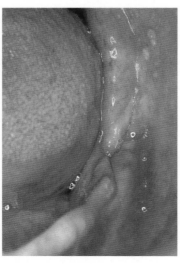

Follow-up

Sutures are removed and the incision has healed satisfactorily when reviewed at 7 days.

6 Third molar removal

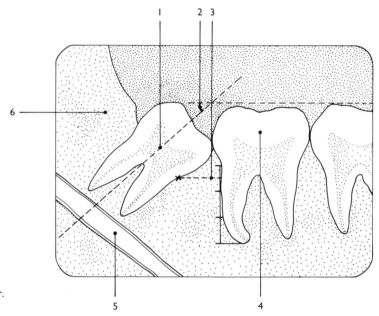

Radiographic assessment of a third molar. Numbers refer to headings below.

Radiographic assessment of third molars

Accurate pre-operative assessment of third molars by means of a good quality radiograph is crucial to successful surgery, and sadly so often neglected. These notes have been included to highlight its importance. The following should be considered:

1. Third molar form

Crown

- Size
- Shape
- Caries status

Root

- Size
- Shape—bulbous or tapered
  —curvature
  —parallelism
  —apical form
- Number

2. Angulation

- Angle of mean long axis of the third molar to the 'occlusal plane'. (This can only be an estimate, since accurate geometrical construction would be tedious and unnecessary, and the 'occlusal plane' is not a straight line.)

● Described as mesio-angular (acute angle), vertical (right angle), disto-angular (obtuse angle), or horizontal (parallel).

3. Depth

● Conveniently defined by referring the standard mesial point of elevation of the third molar to the root of the second molar. The mesial point of application is seen on the radiograph as the enamel–cementum junction, and this can be related by eye to the upper, middle or lower third of the distal root of the second molar.

4. Second molar

Crown

● Size
● Shape
● Caries status and restorations

Root

● Size
● Shape
● Number

5. Inferior dental canal

The relationship of the inferior dental canal to the third molar roots must be established by adequate radiography so that any potential injury to the neurovascular bundle can be anticipated and discussed fully with the patient. The radiographic image of the canal is produced by the cortical lining of the bony tube that contains the soft tissue. When one or other margin of the tube is absent, then the linear image is interrupted as it crosses the root. In the rare case of true perforation, both lines are interrupted and there is a dark band of reduced radiopacity across the root, produced by relative absence of root dentine in this plane. There is also an apparent narrowing or constriction of the white

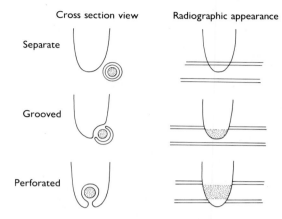

Radiographic assessment of the inferior dental canal.

linear outline as it meets a grooved or perforated root. Deviation of the normally smoothly curved outline of the canal is also common when there is a true relationship to the root.

6. Distal bone level

The exact relationship of the distal bone to the crown of the impacted tooth is important because clearance in this area is required to upright or deliver the tooth. Because of the superimposition of the radiodense inner and outer cortical plates, even a large distal defect may be difficult to detect, especially when pericoronal infection has destroyed its cortical surface. However, a healthy or even a cystic follicle will produce a clear outline. The relationship of the distal bone should be confirmed by probing prior to elevation of a partially erupted tooth.

Partially-erupted mesio-angular lower third molar

PMcD, a 17-year-old student, had an episode of pericoronitis related to his lower left third molar, which was treated successfully with penicillin and with warm saline mouthwashes. The treatment plan involved extraction of this tooth, and prophylactic removal of the other third molars. He agreed to have the teeth removed, one side at a time, under local anaesthesia. The symptomatic side, the left, was treated first, but the operation on the right side is illustrated.

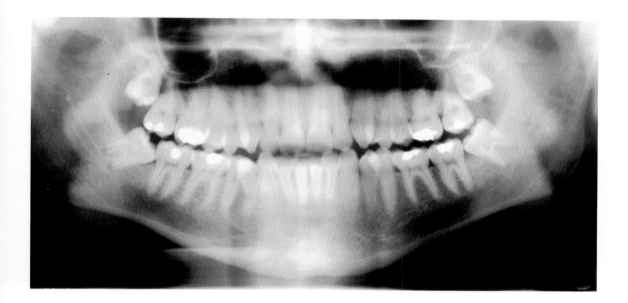

Radiographic assessment

The lower right third molar has a moderately large, sound crown, and the roots are straight with a large interradicular space. There is marked mesio-angular inclination, and the mesial point of application is level with the upper third of the second molar root. The second molar roots are tapered and its crown is intact, apart from a small buccal amalgam filling. The inferior dental canal is close to the mesial root apex and the distal bone is level with the neck of the third molar. Since the tooth will be delivered upwards and backwards, pressure from the mesial root on the canal contents is unlikely.

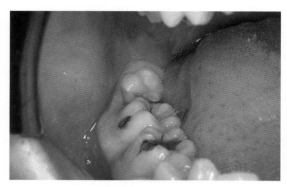

Operation

Operation site

The partially-erupted third molar is surrounded by a gingival cuff of variable thickness, free of inflammation. The mesial part of the crown is directly in contact with the distal surface of the second molar crown.

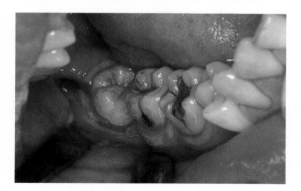

Incision

The first incision is made to bisect the gingival margin distally, and the second started with the blade against the distal surface of the second molar, cutting across the attached gingivae and turning forward for a short distance into the sulcus, to end level with the mesial surface of the second molar. No attempt is made to incise around the crown of the third molar since the tissues will strip off easily.

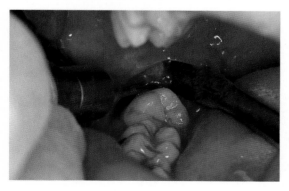

Reflection

The flap is reflected with a Howarth's periosteal elevator, starting in the mesial incision. A second Howarth's can be used to hold the flap open while the distal tissues are reflected cleanly off the bone. It is essential that the subperiosteal plane is identified, especially over the internal oblique ridge distally to the third molar crown, so that a guard instrument can be inserted to protect the lingual tissues during distal bone cutting.

Bone removal

The tooth is in clear view and a natural mesial point of application already exists. It is therefore necessary only to relieve the impaction by removal of a gutter of bone distally so that the tooth may be uprighted.

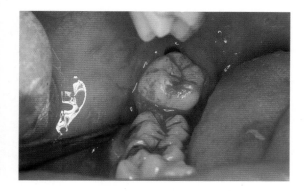

Elevation and delivery

A Warwick-James' elevator is inserted mesially and turned in order to upright and elevate the tooth. If necessary, it can also be elevated using buccal application at the bifurcation of the roots. Only moderate force should be used. If there is resistance, then further distal bone removal will overcome the problem.

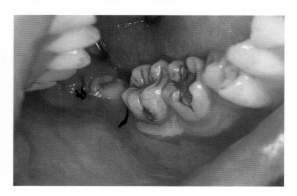

Socket

The socket is free of debris, and the flap lies in position.

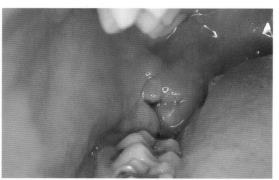

Closure

Two sutures are used. The first advances the mesial corner across the socket, and the second closes the distal incision.

Follow-up

A week later the wound has closed, though the tissue margins are still oedematous. Frequent warm saline mouthbaths are advised and, if necessary, a disposable syringe may be given to the patient to be used for irrigation.

Unerupted mesio-angular impaction

DK, a 21-year-old apprentice joiner, complained of numbness in the right lower jaw. No explanation could be found, but he was advised to have the unerupted right lower third molar removed, in case the impacted tooth might be producing pressure on the inferior dental nerve in an attempt to erupt. Grossly carious lower first molars had been removed 4 years before, but this had not avoided third molar impaction.

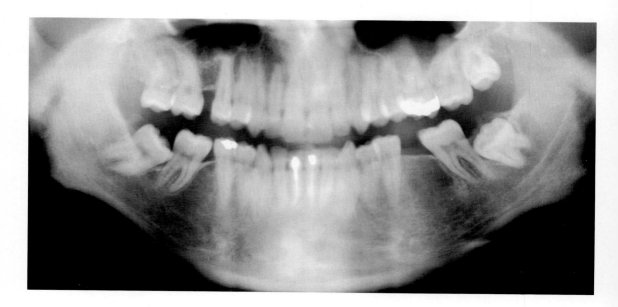

Radiographic assessment

The large lower right third molar has tapered roots with a tendency to distal curvature, which is more pronounced in the mesial root. There is marked mesio-angular inclination, and the mesial point of elevation is level with the middle third of the distal root of the second molar. The second is the only erupted molar in this quadrant, its roots are of normal size and shape, and its crown is caries-free. The inferior dental canal is not clearly demarcated, but it seems to run a safe distance beneath the root apices. The distal bone level is at the neck of the tooth, but there is a faint radiopacity which suggests a broad, bony dish around the crown. This impression is strengthened when the other side is examined, as it shows a similar feature more clearly.

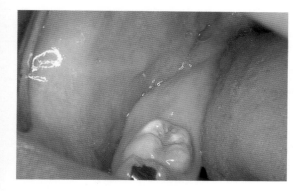

Operation

Operation site

The impacted tooth is covered by a bulky, fibrous mass which will be easy to incise cleanly and will form a robust flap. A faint distal groove can be seen.

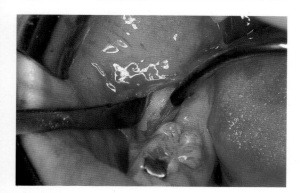

Incision

The incision runs from the distal groove, across the fibrous pad, to the disto-buccal corner of the second molar. The second incision is made at a right angle to the first, and then carried across the attached gingivae to finish in a short, shallow forward curve.

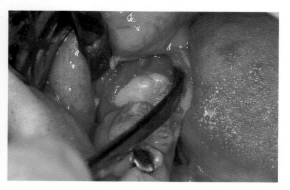

Reflection

The flap is reflected buccally with a Howarth's periosteal elevator. The clean, white bony surface can easily be seen as the sucker mops up the bleeding from a soft tissue tag.

Further reflection distally and lingually exposes the crown of the tooth which is surrounded by a bulky, soft tissue follicle.

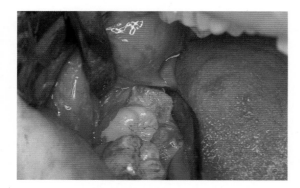

The follicular tissue has been removed and the extent of the bony crypt can be seen. The large lingual shelf is a bizarre and unusual feature of this case.

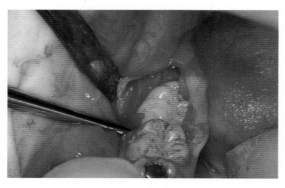

Elevation and delivery

A straight Warwick-James' elevator is inserted mesially and the tooth is easily displaced upwards.

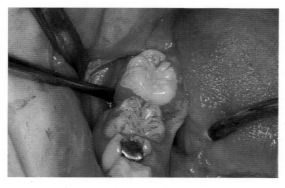

It is pushed up further by inserting the same instrument into the bifurcation and applying leverage against the buccal bone.

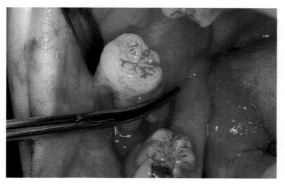

The tooth is lifted out by grasping the attached soft tissue with artery forceps—a convenient way of removing both at once.

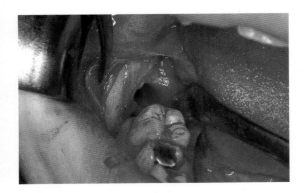

Socket

The lingual bony excrescence is nibbled smooth with rongeurs and the socket aspirated clean of debris.

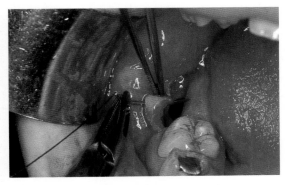

Closure

The corner of the flap is drawn across to the lingual side.

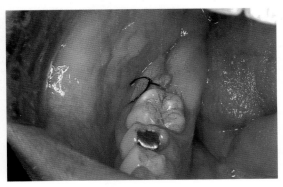

A single suture holds the flap in good position.

Follow-up

Healing was uneventful. The original complaint of numbness had disappeared by the time the patient came to surgery.

Horizontal impaction

AD, a 29-year-old electrician, presented with painful inflammation of the operculum overlying an impacted lower right third molar. The upper right third molar, which was biting on the swollen operculum, was extracted. The pocket beneath the operculum was flushed with aqueous chlorhexidine (0.2 per cent). Aqueous iodine was applied and a 5-day course of metronidazole prescribed (200 mg, three times daily). When reviewed at 7 days, the acute condition had settled and an appointment was arranged for removal of the lower third molar. The patient was warned of the possibility of nerve damage, and the warning recorded in the case notes.

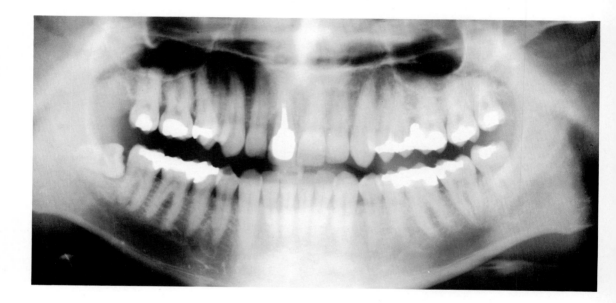

Radiographic assessment

The lower right third molar is of normal size and shape, and is in horizontal impaction with the mesial cusps almost in contact with the tooth in front. The mesial point of application is level with the midpoint of the distal root of the second molar. The outline of the inferior dental canal crosses the tip of the mesial root of the third molar, but there is nothing to indicate grooving or perforation. The periapical view, as is often the case with horizontal impactions, does not extend far enough distally to show the whole of the root and this important relationship. If no other technique is available, it may be possible to gain the patient's co-operation in repeating the view with a film placed more distally than before. This co-operation is vital, since the more posterior placement is uncomfortable. An alternative is to use a film holder or an artery clip.

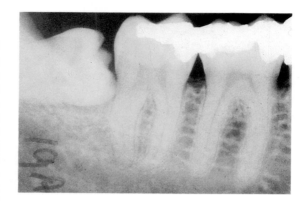

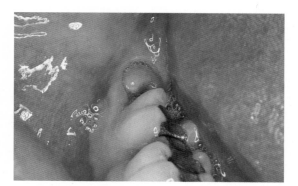

Operation

Operation site

The tooth is partially erupted, with the disto-buccal cusp visible. The distal gingival margin can easily be bisected by an incision from the distal groove, and the buccal gingival roll is thick and will form a good corner for advancing across the socket. The distal surface of the second molar is apparently intact and unweakened by caries or restoration.

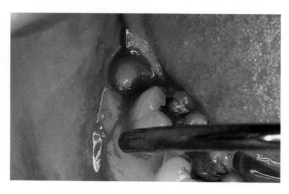

Incision

The incision was made as planned. Note the angle at which the incision crosses the attached gingivae.

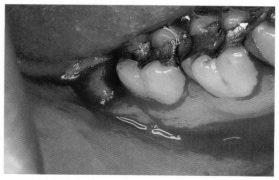

Minor bleeding is often encountered from small vessels cut at the end of the relieving incision. This can be minimized by keeping the angle of the relieving incision as flat as possible. In any case the bleeding is usually transient and stops when the flap is retracted.

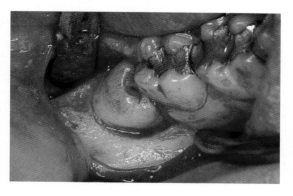

Reflection

A generous exposure has been achieved and, when the remnants of follicle are removed, a more precise appraisal can be made of the angulation of the tooth and its relationship to the bone and the second molar.

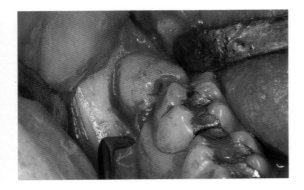

Point of application

The point of a curved Warwick-James' elevator is inserted to confirm that a point of application can be reached. Even a minor degree of movement at this stage will be helpful, but the force should be applied judiciously.

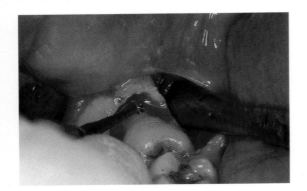

Bone removal

A gutter has been created on the buccal and distal side by cutting to a depth of about half the root length, using the root itself as a cutting guide. Elevation is tried and is partially successful, but the crown is held by the disto-lingual bone.

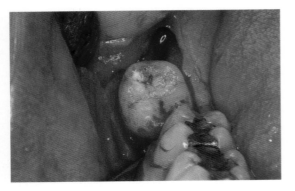

The crucial disto-lingual corner is now cut through, taking care to cut out through to the lingually placed Howarth's periosteal elevator, which acts as a guard and prevents damage to the lingual tissues, including especially the lingual nerve.

Elevation

The tooth can now be uprighted and is free for delivery. Caries and calculus deposits can be seen on the occlusal surface.

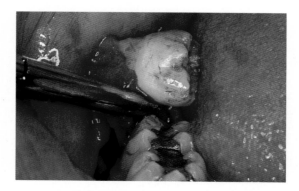

Delivery

The follicular soft tissue tag is grasped with a haemostat and used to lift out the tooth. A loosened tooth will always come away with the follicle, but the reverse is not reliably true.

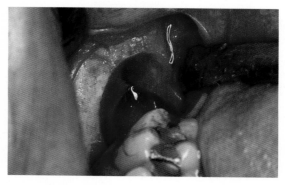

The socket is clean but must be checked for calculus or other debris lying in the blind spot distal to the second molar.

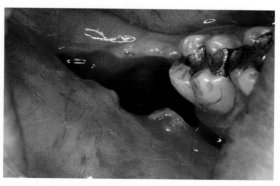

Closure

The soft tissues fall back naturally into position.

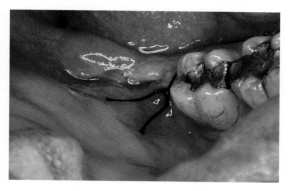

Closure is simply achieved with a single suture.

Follow-up

The wound healed satisfactorily, and the postoperative course was trouble-free.

Disto-angular impaction

MH, a 43-year-old housewife, had suffered repeated episodes of painful pericoronitis associated with her lower right third molar. She had been treated previously with antiseptic irrigation and antimicrobials, and advised to have the tooth removed. When examined, the soft tissue overlying the tooth was thickened and scarred, and the upper right third molar was biting on it. Removal of both teeth was advised, and a warning of possible nerve damage was given and recorded. The patient was willing to have the extraction under local anaesthesia.

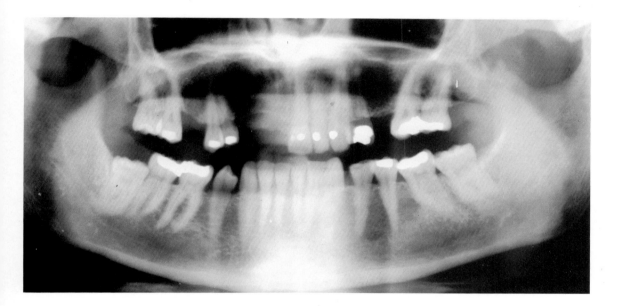

Radiographic assessment

The lower right third molar is large and the fused roots have an apical extension with a marked distal hook. The inclination is disto-angular and the mesial point of application is level with the midpoint of the distal root of the second molar. This tooth has tapered roots and its crown is intact distally. The distal bone is level with the tip of the distal cusp, but there is a generous follicular space. The outline of the inferior dental nerve canal crosses the apex and the apical hook. The relationship is best seen on the orthopantomograph, since the periapical film was not placed distally enough to show the full extent of the root. This radiograph shows how easy it is to miss a narrow apical extension, even on a well-positioned film.

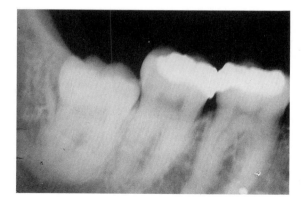

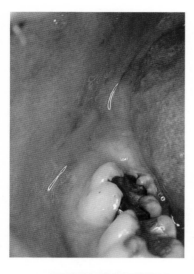

Operation

Operation site

The distal groove is clearly seen in this case. The tooth is completely unerupted and the distal surface of the second molar is sound.

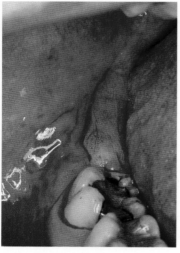

Incision

The incision is placed in the groove, with the relieving branch running across the attached gingivae and the external oblique ridge, then forward to end level with the first and second molar interspace.

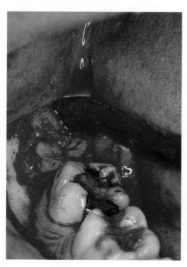

Reflection

The occlusal surface of the third molar is revealed and a Howarth's periosteal elevator is pushed subperiosteally over the internal oblique ridge at the disto-lingual corner.

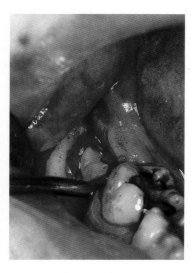

Point of application

A straight Warwick-James' elevator is inserted mesially, and some upward displacement achieved.

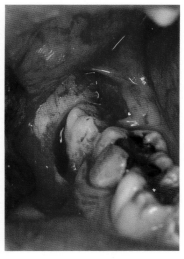

The crown is impinging on the distal bone. Elevation moves the crown backwards, as well as upwards, because of the root curvature.

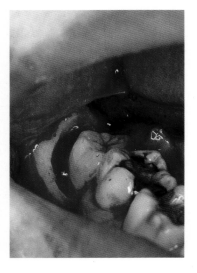

Bone removal

Bone has been removed to deepen the buccal gutter and relieve the impaction distally.

EAST GLAMORGAN GENERAL HOSPITAL
CHURCH VILLAGE. near PONTYPRIDD

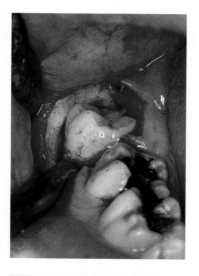

Elevation and delivery

The tooth can now be elevated upwards and backwards out of the socket, using a Cryer's elevator. This has been preferred to a Warwick-James', as the space between the displaced tooth and the second molar is now quite large.

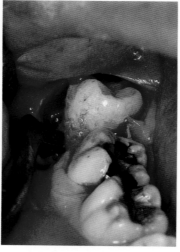

The point of the Cryer's is inserted into the root bifurcation to achieve the final upward displacement and delivery. The loose tooth can be grasped and lifted out with any suitable instrument.

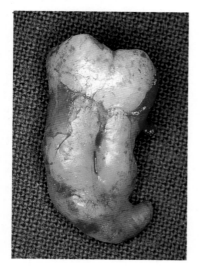

The extracted lower right third molar, viewed from the lingual side, shows the distal hook of the apex and a horizontal groove which may have been related to the inferior dental canal.

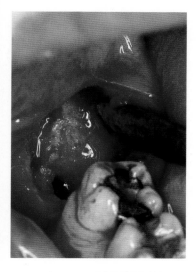

Socket

A clean socket is left, without any debris. None should be expected as the tooth was removed intact, and no bone splintering occurred. The socket surface is already becoming covered with blood coagulum, and this need not be disturbed by flushing.

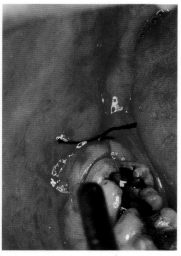

Closure

The incision closes easily with a single suture.

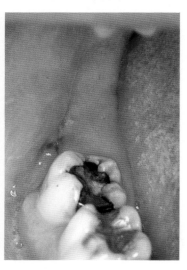

Follow-up

Healing was uneventful, and there was no alteration in nerve function.

Removal of retained unerupted lower third molar

AF, a 31-year-old prisoner, was referred by his prison dentist with a helpful letter which read:

I saw this man a month ago at his insistence and, because he caused a riot, I arranged for him to be brought to my practice where I removed his remaining standing teeth under general anaesthetic. Unfortunately, I was unable to remove the unerupted lower left third molar. I told Mr F that the tooth was still present and most unlikely to cause trouble. However, yesterday, he came to see me again complaining that the tooth was causing trouble and wanting it cut out. As there is considerable bony covering with just the cusps showing above bone level, and the roots appear radiographically to be close to the inferior dental canal, I would be most grateful if you could look at this man and arrange the extraction of the lower left third molar. He is a drug addict and veins in both arms are considerably sclerosed.

The patient complained of a shooting pain on the left side when eating, leading to earache. This symptom is more likely to originate from the temporomandibular joint, but since the provision of dentures would be delayed until the third molar was removed, it was probably the indirect cause of pain. There were no significant findings on examination. In view of his background of drug abuse, a blood sample was taken to exclude hepatitis B infection. This proved to be negative for virus, and positive for antibody. The patient agreed to have the tooth removed under local anaesthesia.

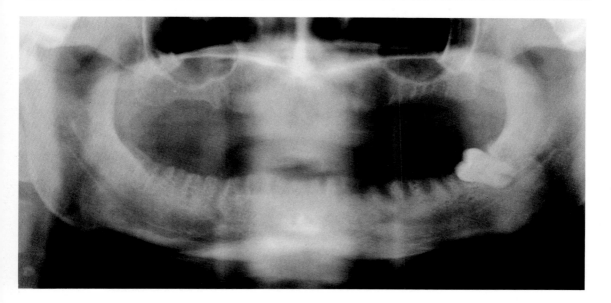

Radiographic assessment

The orthopantomograph shows that there are no other retained teeth or roots. The lower left third molar is normal in size and shape, and lies in mesio-angular inclination with only the distal cusps above the bone level. The follicular space is not obliterated and the distal bone level is just above the distal crown–root junction. The inferior dental canal seems to be in close relationship to the mesial root apex, but the upper white line can just be seen on the original radiograph, and there is no dark banding at the apex. Nevertheless, the patient was warned of the possibility of postoperative lip numbness. The removal of bone in a gutter around the crown should, in any case, allow its elevation away from the apex without tipping the tooth so as to crush the nerve.

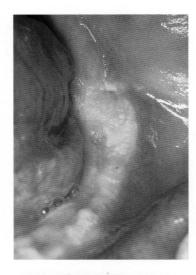

Operation

Site

The extraction sockets have completely healed and there is a broad band of attached gingiva overlying the completely unerupted tooth.

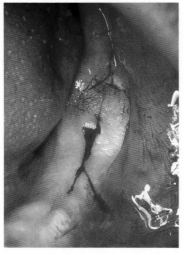

Incision

The main incision is placed just to the buccal side of the crest of the edentulous ridge, from the retromolar area forward to about the first molar area. The relieving incision is made from the first line obliquely forward towards the sulcus. It was intended to run the relieving incision from the anterior limit of the ridge incision, but it has in fact been placed a little distally.

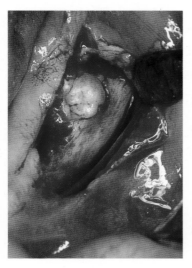

Reflection

The flap is reflected with a Howarth's periosteal elevator and the external oblique ridge can be seen clearly.

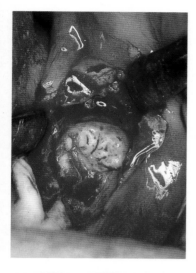

The flap must be reflected cleanly over the internal oblique ridge, distally and lingually, since blind cutting in this area can endanger the lingual nerve.

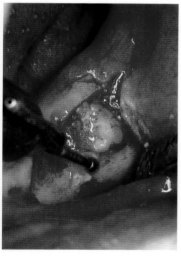

Bone removal

Using a small rosehead bur, bone is removed to form a deep, narrow gutter around the buccal and mesial sides of the crown.

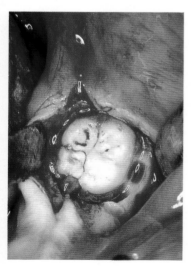

The entire circumference of the crown has been cleared.

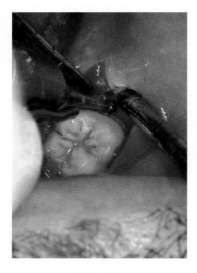

The crucial distal bony gutter is made, with a Howarth's inserted to guard the lingual soft tissues.

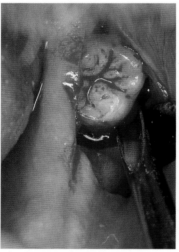

Elevation

The tooth is now easily elevated, using a large Coupland's chisel inserted, buccally and mesially, into the gutter, and rotated to impinge on the tooth surface and drive it upwards.

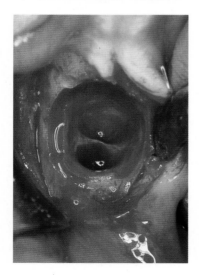

Socket

In cases like these, the socket is in direct line with the operator's vision, so any small apices which may fracture off are easily seen and, with delicate manipulation, it is therefore possible to remove them.

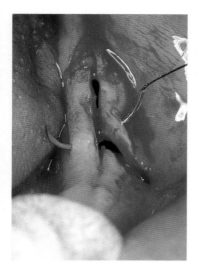

Closure

The first suture is placed across the corner of the flap that was deliberately created at the time of incision to aid relocation.

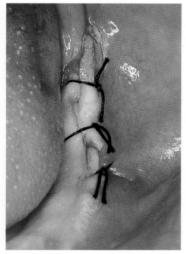

Two further sutures close the distal limb.

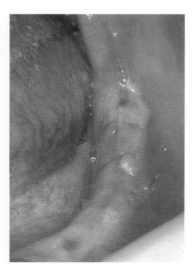

Follow-up

Sutures are removed at 1 week, and the wound has healed very satisfactorily. The patient was referred back to the prison dentist for provision of dentures.

Removal of unerupted upper third molar

AH, a 19-year-old dental surgery assistant, had suffered an episode of pericoronitis related to the lower right third molar, and had in the past undergone orthodontic treatment to align the upper canines following surgical exposure. The third molars were all completely unerupted and their removal was indicated. Despite having one congenitally-absent kidney, she was in good health and agreed to have the teeth removed, one side at a time, under local anaesthesia.

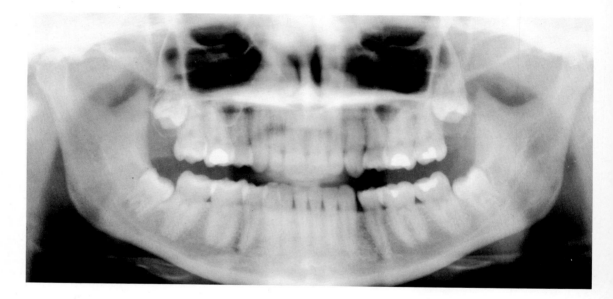

Radiographic assessment

The upper right third molar is of normal size and shape and has an incompletely formed root. It is surrounded by follicle and lies in a spacious bony crypt. It has a slight disto-angular inclination, and is deeply placed with the mesial elevation point at the level of the apices of the upper second molar. The maxillary sinus is large and adjoins the unerupted tooth.

The upper left third molar is in a similar position, but even higher, and there are two mesio-angular lowers present.

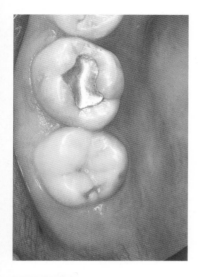

Operation

The first three and penultimate photographs have been taken using a mirror and are printed inverted, so as to relate more easily to the other photographs in the sequence.

Operation site

The second molar has an intact distal surface and there is no sign of eruption of the third molar.

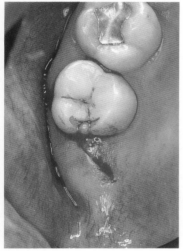

Incision

The incision runs in a straight line from the palatal side of the tuberosity, obliquely forward at a tangent to the disto-buccal corner of the second molar, and up across the buccal attached gingivae towards the sulcus.

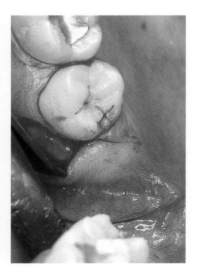

Reflection

The flap is raised with a Howarth's periosteal elevator, starting anteriorly and working around the maxillary tuberosity beneath the mucoperiosteum.

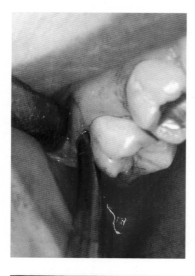

Bone removal

The thin buccal plate of bone overlying the tooth follicle is easily flaked off by inserting a Coupland's chisel and levering it outwards.

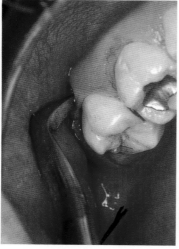

Elevation and delivery

A Cryer's elevator is used to lever the tooth downwards, backwards and outwards so as to displace it from its crypt. The sharp point can be used to force a point of application, mesially.

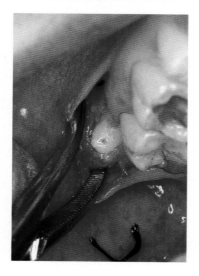

When loosened, the tooth is lifted out with a convenient instrument – in this case, a pair of artery forceps.

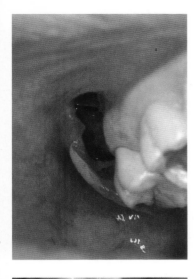

Closure

The wound is gaping open and requires to be sutured to appose the edges. In the majority of cases, an upper third molar wound would lie together well enough without suturing.

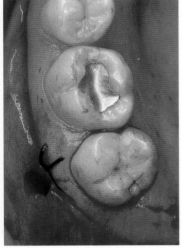

The first suture reconstitutes the buccal gingival margin.

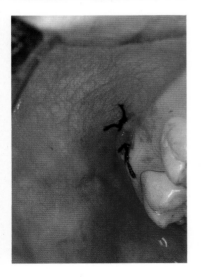

As the buccal end of the incision is still gaping and bleeding, a second suture has been inserted there.

Follow-up

The wound healed perfectly.

7   Endodontic surgery

Apicectomy of upper right central incisor

KF, a 22-year-old electrician, complained of pain, constant over three days, in the upper right anterior region. A small pustule could be seen in the sulcus between the upper right central and lateral incisors. A periapical radiograph showed a large, diffuse radiolucent area at the apex of the central incisor with destruction of the apical lamina dura. Involvement of the lateral incisor was suspected, but the tooth responded normally to vitality tests. Apicectomy and retrograde root-filling of the upper right central incisor were advised, and an appointment made for treatment under local anaesthesia.

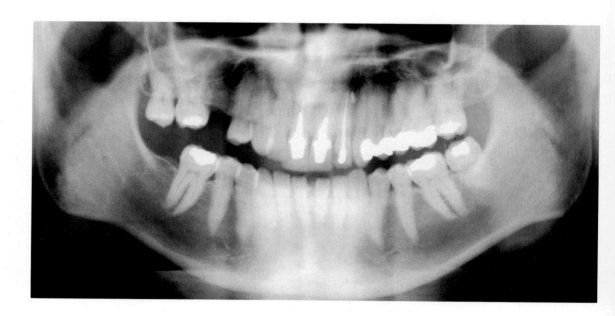

Radiographic assessment

The orthopantomograph shows that both the upper central incisors have been root-filled and post-crowned, and that there are no other problems requiring surgery. The apparent periapical radiolucency, related to the over-filled upper left lateral incisor, was not confirmed in a periapical view, which showed no evidence of active disease about the apices of either left incisor. The periapical view of the upper right incisors shows the root filling in the central incisor to be well short of the apex. There is a loss of lamina dura distally from the apical third of the root, and an ill-defined radiolucent area extending to the root of the lateral incisor. The root canal of the lateral incisor has a sharp distal curvature and the lamina dura at its apex seems intact.

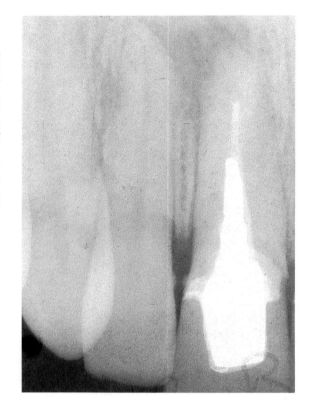

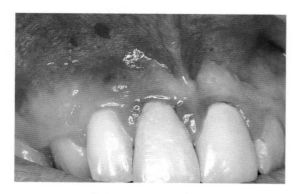

Operation

Operation site

The gingival condition about the crowned upper central incisors is poor and the labial fraenal attachment is close to the papilla between these teeth. No sinus can be seen.

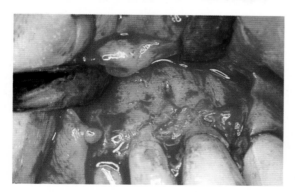

Incision

The incision commences in the sulcus on the left side of the fraenum, and the cut is made towards the mesial surface of the left central incisor, so as to include the interdental papilla in the flap. The tip of the scalpel blade is run round the gingival margins of the upper right incisors and canine.

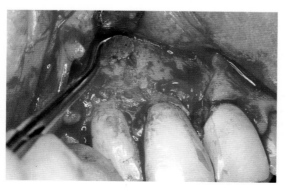

Reflection

The flap is reflected using two Howarth's periosteal elevators. The defective labial bony support of the central incisor can be clearly seen. There is a small bony notch which probably marks the former exit of a discharging sinus.

Bone removal

A Mitchell's trimmer is used to chip away the thin, undermined bony plate overlying the periapical granuloma.

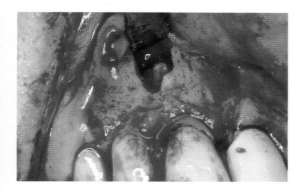

The granulation tissue has been curetted away and the apex is in clear view.

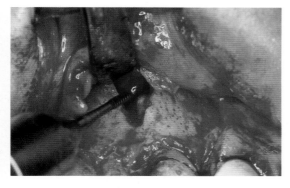

Apical section

A fine flat fissure bur is used to cut across the root and sever the apex.

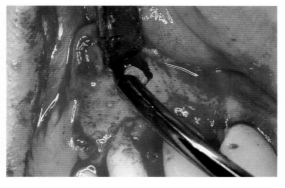

The apex is removed with the sucker tip.

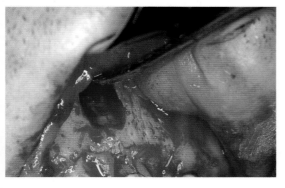

The cut surface is angled so that the root canal opening can be seen.

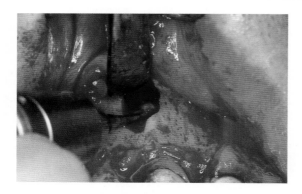

Retrograde root-filling

A small rosehead bur is used to cut an undercut cavity.

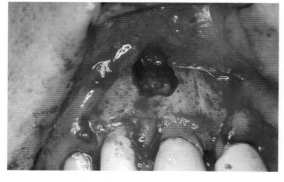

The prepared cavity.

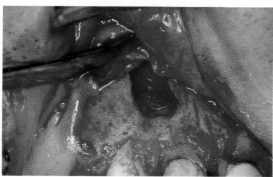

Amalgam is placed to seal the end of the root canal.

Closure

The flap is repositioned and sutured into position. The first suture replaces the interdental papilla between the central incisors, and the second replaces the papilla between the central and lateral incisors. The third suture is placed in the sulcus across the relieving limb.

Follow-up

The tissues healed well, but the symptoms recurred. A repeat procedure, performed a few months later, resolved the problem.

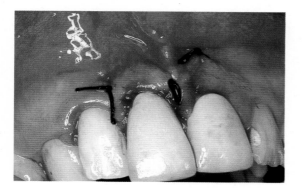

8 Orthodontic surgery

Upper labial fraenectomy

In the case of JC, a 16-year-old schoolgirl, the presence of the large fraenum was thought to be contributing to the persistence of the upper midline diastema. The patient agreed to have the fraenum excised under local anaesthesia.

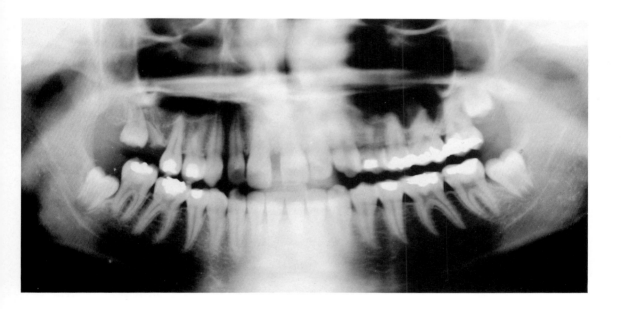

Radiographic assessment

An orthopantomograph (see page 61) taken at the beginning of orthodontic treatment, a year before referral, showed a high caries rate with active lesions in at least two molars and a retained root in the upper right molar region. The anterior occlusal film confirms that there was no evidence of a mid-line supernumerary tooth, and the upper central incisors were of a normal shape and structure.

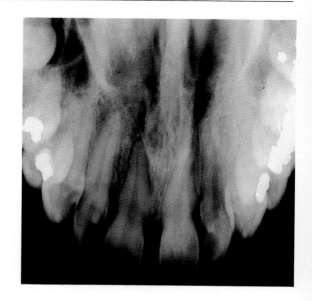

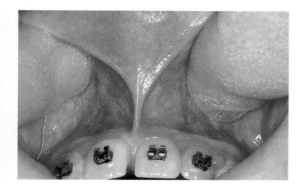

Operation

Operation site

The attachment of the fraenum is demonstrated by traction, with a finger in the sulcus on either side. The co-operation of an assistant, using the fingers of both hands to grasp and evert the lip firmly in this way, is essential both to provide retraction and to help reduce bleeding by occlusion of the labial vessels.

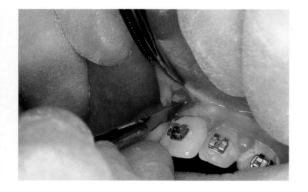

Excision

The fraenum is grasped in a curved haemostat.

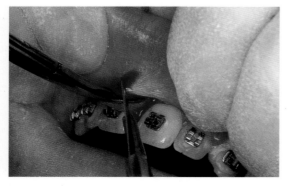

It is released by an incision on either side of its base.

Excision is completed by running the scalpel edge down the back of the haemostat.

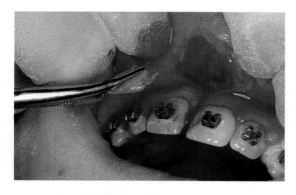

The excised tissue is removed.

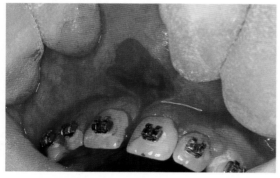

A diamond-shaped defect is left.

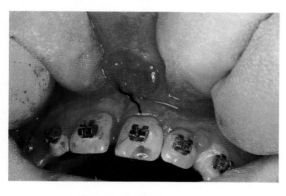

Closure

The first suture is placed at the base of the defect so as to draw in the wound edges and tether them together to the periosteum at the depth of the sulcus.

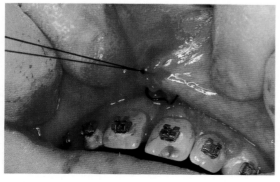

Further sutures close the labial part of the defect. The alveolar side of the wound may be dressed with a periodontal pack if the exposed area is large or if the bleeding is troublesome.

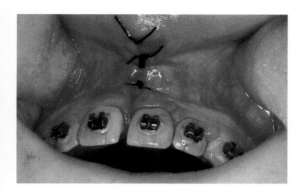

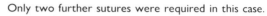
Only two further sutures were required in this case.

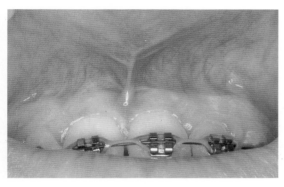

Follow-up

Three months later the wound has healed well and the mid-line diastema has almost closed. The small residual scar is more prominent in the photograph than in reality!

Removal of supernumerary and exposure of upper lateral incisor

FF, a 12-year-old schoolgirl, presented with mild upper arch crowding and failure of the upper right lateral incisor to erupt. She had a mild Angle Class III malocclusion on a Skeletal Class III base, with slightly higher than average Frankfort-mandibular plane angle. Radiographs showed that the eruption of the upper right lateral incisor was impeded by the presence of a small supernumerary tooth. Since this supernumerary could neither be seen nor palpated buccally, it was deduced that it must lie palatally to the lateral incisor crown. In view of its superficial position, removal under local anaesthesia was offered and accepted. The patient was perfectly fit, although she suffered occasional attacks of asthma, eczema and hay fever.

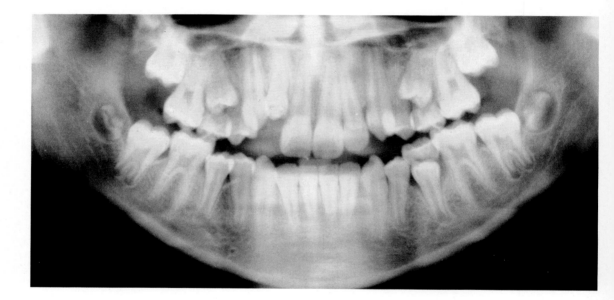

Radiographic assessment

The radiographs show a crowded mixed dentition
with noneruption of an otherwise normal-looking
upper right lateral incisor. The supernumerary can
be seen in the orthopantomograph to lie above the
cingulum of the lateral incisor. The occlusal film
shows it clearly, lying obliquely across the crown
of the lateral incisor, with the tip of its crown
placed distally.

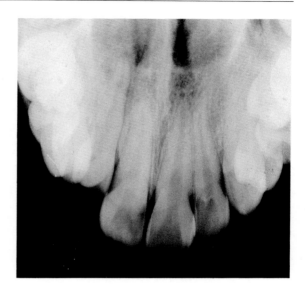

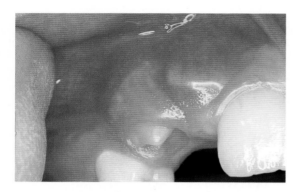

Operation

Site

The incisal edge of the lateral incisor can be clearly seen through the thin, tense overlying mucosa.

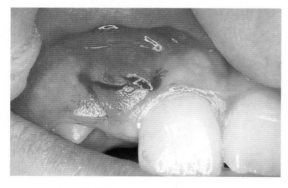

Incision

The incision simply outlines the incisal edge of the lateral incisor.

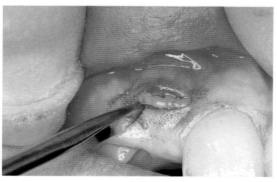

Exposure merely consists of pushing the edge of the thin mucosa apically with a straight Warwick-James' elevator.

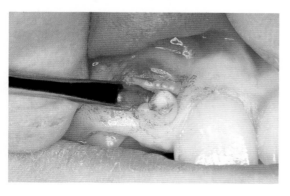

Elevation

The elevator is inserted against the palatal surface of the crown.

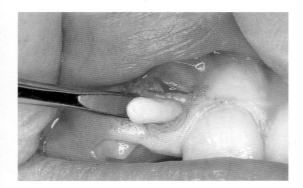

The Warwick-James' pushes the supernumerary mesially and upwards out of its crypt.

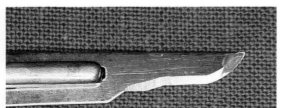

The small conical tooth.

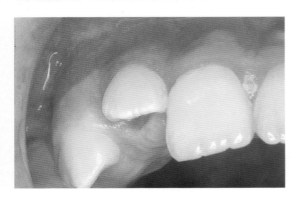

Follow-up

The upper second primary molars and first premolars were extracted and, 3 months later, an upper removal orthodontic appliance was used to retract the erupting right upper canine and to make space for the lateral incisor to come into position.

Exposure of upper canine

MD, a 13-year-old schoolgirl, presented with an unerupted misplaced upper left canine. She had a crowded upper arch and a shift of the midline to the right with an Angle Class I incisor relationship on a Skeletal Class I base. Removal of the retained but mobile upper left deciduous canine and the four second premolars was advised. The first stage was to be the removal of the deciduous canine and exposure of the permanent successor. The patient agreed to have this done under local anaesthesia.

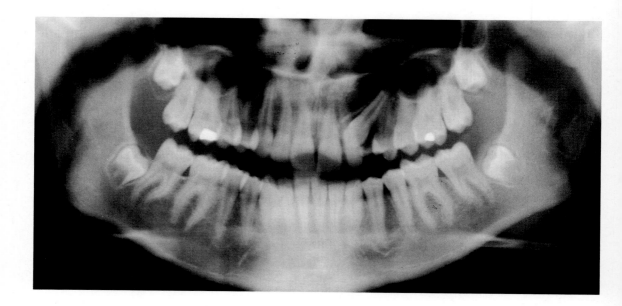

Radiographic assessment

The patient had a full adult dentition and one retained deciduous canine, of which hardly any root remains. She is almost caries-free, but there appears to be a recurrent lesion beneath the amalgam in the upper right first molar. The upper left permanent canine is tilted, with the crown overlapping the lateral incisor. The periapical film shows the tooth to be of normal shape and size, and confirms the advanced resorption of the deciduous tooth. The vertex occlusal film clearly shows that the tip of the crown is placed palatally to the lateral incisor.

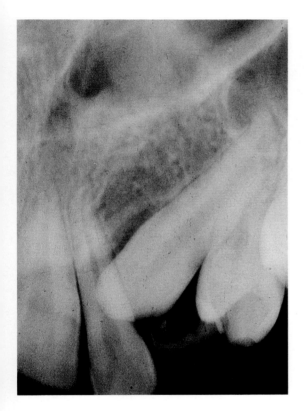

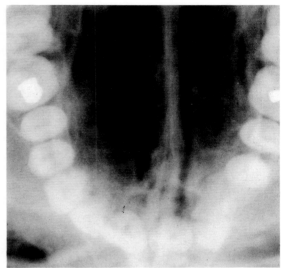

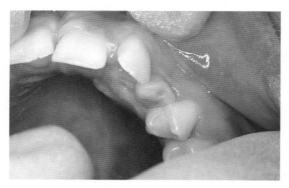

Operation

Operation site

The fractured upper left lateral incisor and the retained deciduous canine can be clearly seen, and there is a 'bump' palatally overlying the unerupted tooth. The exposure can be achieved within the attached gingival tissue.

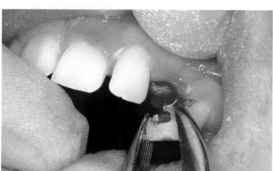

Extraction

The deciduous canine is simply removed with forceps.

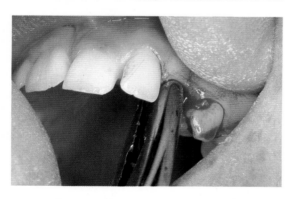

Exposure

The first bite of tissue over the crown is removed with rongeurs.

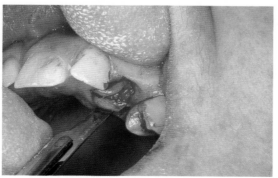

The excision is completed with a scalpel.

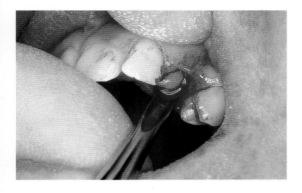

The gingival tissues are pushed back from the newly-exposed crown with a Coupland's chisel. This will also create some space in the bone which is required for the tooth to erupt.

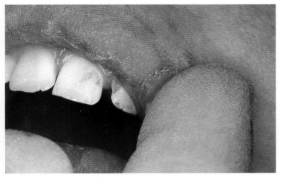

Dressing

The lips are lubricated with petroleum jelly to prevent the resin from the pack sticking to the lips and the skin of the face.

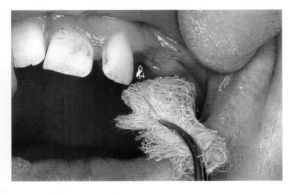

The 1 cm ribbon gauze pack has been soaked in iodoform and blotted dry on a swab.

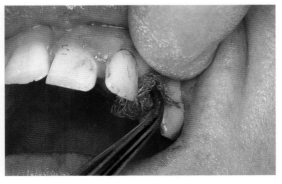

The pack is placed over the exposed crown and tucked into position beneath the soft tissues buccally and palatally.

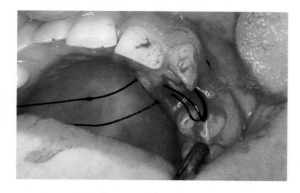

The pack has proved unstable without support, so a mattress suture is inserted across the defect and loops drawn up in the central portion.

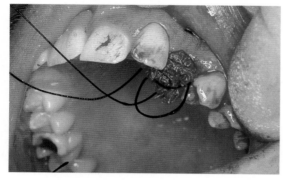

The pack is then re-inserted beneath the loops, which are drawn tight one at a time by traction on the loose ends.

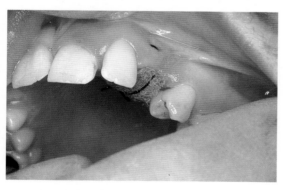

The suture is tied and cut (such sutures are more usually tied on the buccal side).

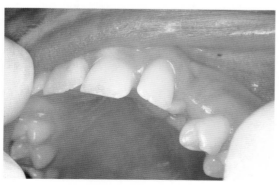

Follow-up

The pack was removed in 7 days and healing was excellent. If exposure is wider and more raw surface is exposed, then the pack may be left in position for 10–14 days. A bracket or attachment can be cemented to the exposed crown surface and, after initial healing, traction can be applied to guide or accelerate eruption.

9 Prosthodontic surgery

Smoothing of edentulous ridge

MMcM, a 43-year-old housewife, complained of pain beneath her lower denture in the right anterior region, which persisted in spite of adjustment of the denture. No obvious localizing cause could be found on clinical or radiographic examination, and there was generalized rather than focal tenderness. It was decided by a colleague that the area should be explored under local anaesthesia, and the underlying bony ridge smoothed. The operation was advised in the hope of a favourable outcome and in response to the patient's wish for some positive action. Had the surgical intervention been other than trivial, it would not have been agreed. Perhaps a more thorough search for a psychogenic cause of the symptoms would have been fruitful.

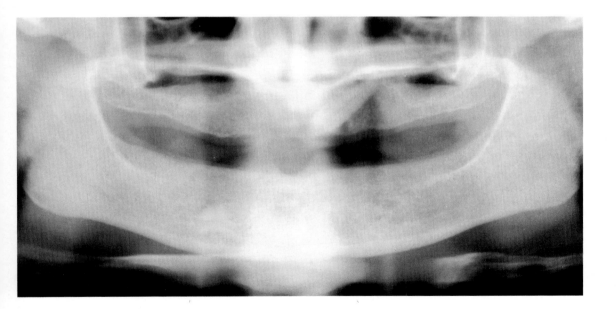

Radiographic assessment

The orthopantomograph (see page 75) shows the patient to be truly edentulous apart from a retained unerupted upper left canine, which lies beneath the margin of the bony ridge and demonstrates no related pathological changes. The lower anterior region appears to be perfectly smooth and regular in outline on this film. The more detailed periapical view contributes little more, other than to exclude definitely the presence of any root fragments.

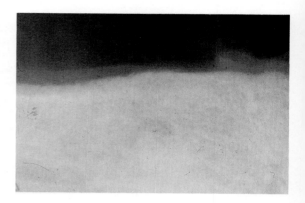

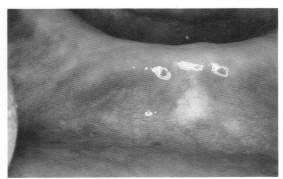

Operation

Operation site

The edentulous lower ridge looks quite normal. The central blanched area is produced by traction on the lip and does not indicate the presence of a bony lump!

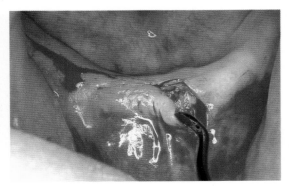

Incision

The incision runs just buccally to the crest of the ridge from the molar region to just across the midline, where it is continued in a short-angled relieving limb.

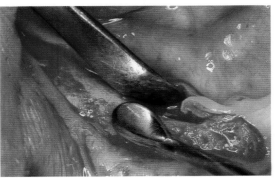

Reflection

The friable tissues are reflected using the curette end of a Mitchell's trimmer initially, followed by the insertion of a Howarth's periosteal elevator.

Bone-smoothing

When exposed buccally and lingually, the ridge is inspected for abnormalities of shape and surface, and is smoothed with a small bone file.

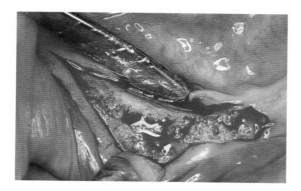

The cortical crest of the ridge after smoothing.

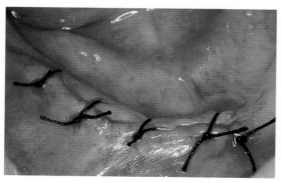

Closure

The wound is closed with five sutures, the first being inserted at the anterior corner to relocate the flap.

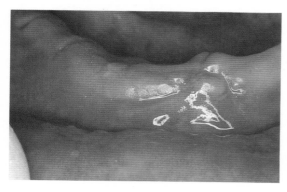

Follow-up

Sutures were removed a week later, and the wound has healed well. The patient was unavailable for further follow-up.

Surgical removal of fibrous tuberosity

HM, a 45-year-old perfume consultant, required reduction of a large, flabby left maxillary tuberosity, prior to the construction of a new upper denture. She had no symptoms, and agreed to have the surgery under local anaesthesia.

Radiographic assessment

The orthopantomograph shows the patient to be completely edentulous. The outline of a large, left maxillary tuberosity can be made out, and it appears to consist entirely of fibrous tissue. The shape and extent of the underlying bone is quite symmetrical.

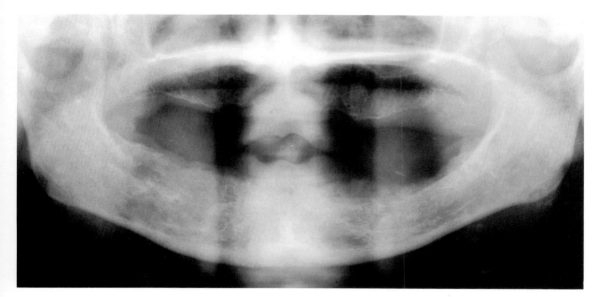

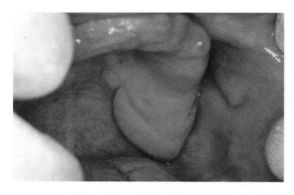

Operation

Operation site

The left maxillary tuberosity is mobile and deeply undercut.

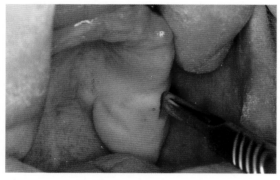

Incision

A Y-shaped incision is made, commencing from about the second molar region and diverging buccally and palatally.

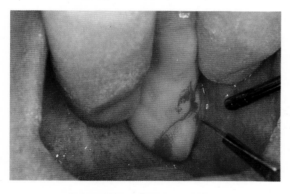

A wedge of tissue is demarcated for excision.

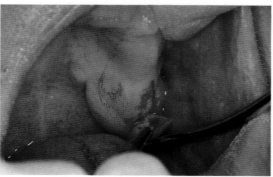

The wedge is cut free at its base and excised.

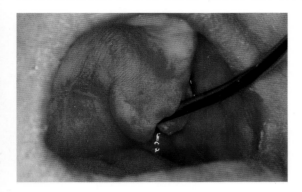

The edges of the defect are undermined by cutting into them with the scalpel so as to mobilize them for closure.

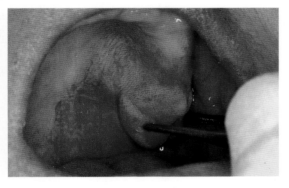

The flaps are brought together with tissue forceps to check the extent of reduction obtained.

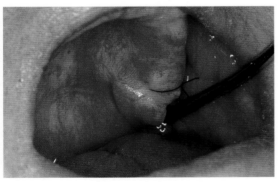

Closure

Sutures are placed so as to draw the wound edges together into the best shape which can be achieved.

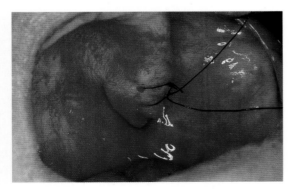

The position of the flaps is controlled by careful suture placement.

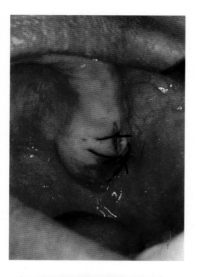

Deep bites of tissue are taken, and the sutures are placed under slight tension. Further undermining cuts may be needed if the tension is judged to be excessive.

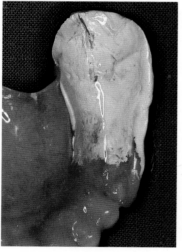

Dressing

A dressing of zinc-oxide/eugenol paste is applied to the denture to cover the wound and support the tissues in the new position.

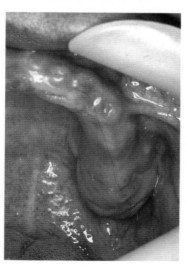

Follow-up

Sutures were removed 7 days later and the initial healing was satisfactory.

Excision of denture-induced hyperplasia

IL, a 54-year-old houswife, complained of a 'piece of skin' growing out from under her lower denture on the right side. This had been present for a few months and had sometimes become swollen. She had required surgery for a similar problem on the left side approximately 3 years earlier. A large lump of hyperplastic tissue was present, which had a typical bilobed shape with the denture flange in the central cleft. She wished to retain use of the lower denture and so the flange was cut away in the related area to encourage resolution of the local inflammation. An appointment was arranged for excision of the lesion under local anaesthesia.

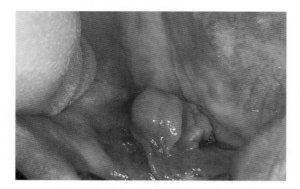

Operation

Operation site

The hyperplastic tissue forms a short thick deeply-clefted lump in the right lower sulcus with a narrow folded extension buccally and forwards.

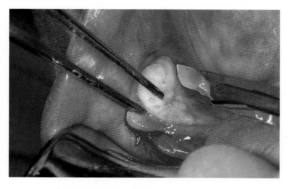

The base was generously infiltrated with local anaesthetic and the lingual fold grasped with tissue forceps. The tissue blanches as the traction reduces its blood supply.

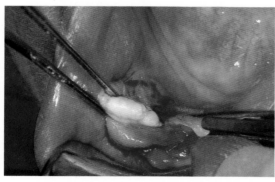

Incision

The soft tissue is held in tension and released by incision at the base.

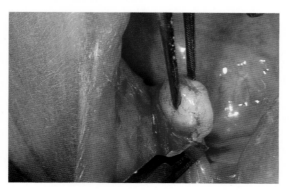

The incision is repeated on the other side.

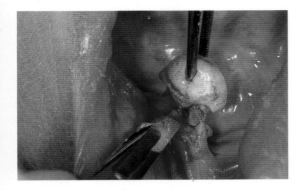

A third sweep of the scalpel separates the lesion completely.

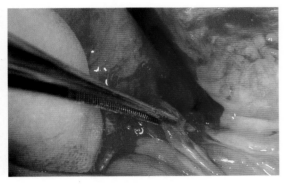

The anterior fold is drawn up.

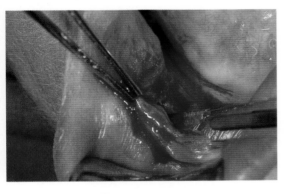

It is incised at the base.

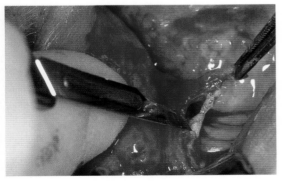

The final strands of fibrous tissue are released.

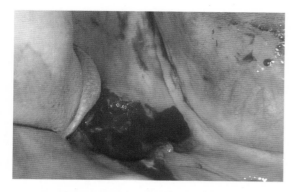

The bleeding comes mostly from capillary oozing.

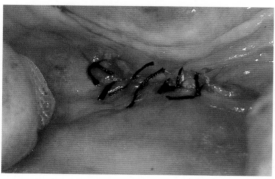

Closure

Bleeding from the raw area is arrested satisfactorily when the edges are drawn together with sutures. Very large areas may require grafting and present a difficult surgical problem.

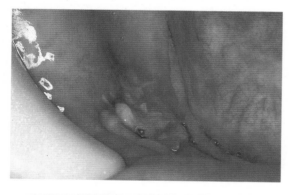

Follow-up

A week after operation, healing is satisfactory.

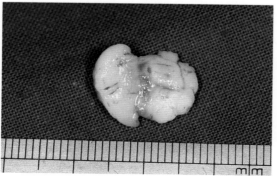

The excised tissue, seen here with a millimetre scale, was sent for histopathological examination.

Pathology report

The pathologist reported that the histology showed features in keeping with the clinical diagnosis of denture-induced hyperplasia.

Removal of unerupted maxillary canine

MG, a 42-year-old housewife, required a replacement upper denture and, as part of the examination and assessment, an orthopantomograph was taken.

An unerupted upper right canine was found to be lying horizontally beneath the upper ridge. In view of the close proximity of the crown to the ridge and its lack of bony cover, removal of the unerupted tooth was advised. The patient agreed to an operation under local anaesthesia.

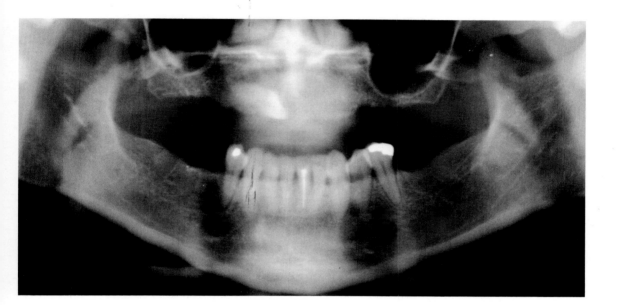

Radiographic assessment

The orthopantomograph (see page 87) demonstrates the presence of the canine and the absence of any other maxillary tooth. The three periapical films demonstrate its size and shape, and show clearly that, in this case, there is no significant apical curvature to complicate extraction.

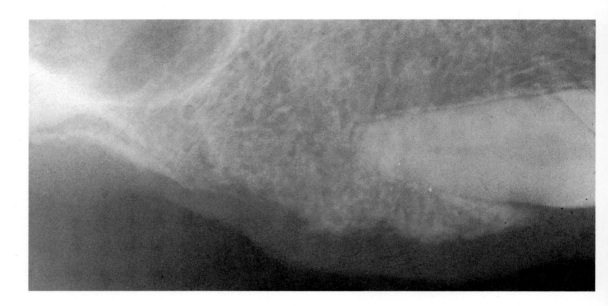

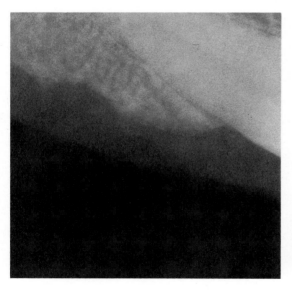

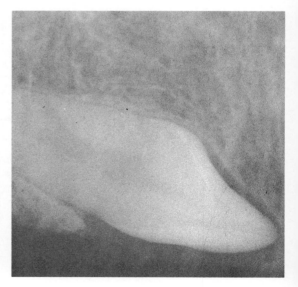

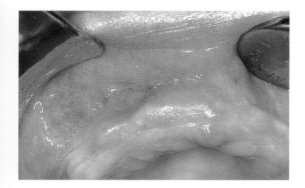

Operation

Operation site

The mucosa is healthy and intact. The tooth crown lies beneath a visible and palpable prominence in the right upper anterior region.

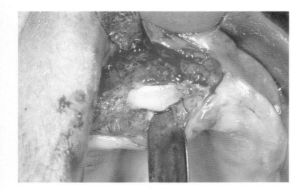

Incision

The incision extends from the right molar region to a relieving limb, just to the left side of the midline. It is placed buccally to the crest of the ridge.

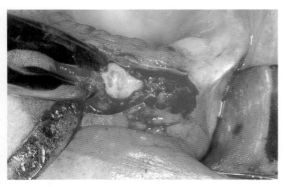

Reflection

The flap is raised with some difficulty due to the complicated mass of fibrous tissue around the crown, but the first cardinal point of the tooth, the distal bulge of the crown, can be seen.

Bone removal

Soft tissue, and then covering bone, is removed gradually with rongeurs to uncover the second point, the tip of the crown. Uncovering the mesial bulge is not necessary, as forceps will be used for extraction.

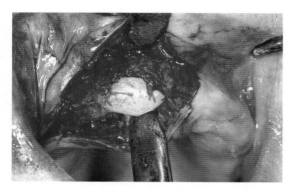

Delivery

The crown is now covered sufficiently for the conventional application of forceps.

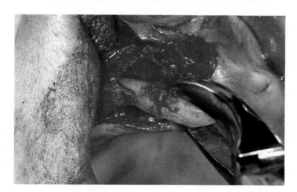

The tooth is grasped in the forceps blades. In these cases, forceps can often be applied mesio-distally to advantage.

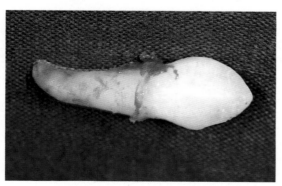

The tooth is delivered easily.

There is minor apical curvature.

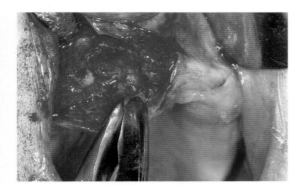

Socket

Soft tissue tags and sharp bony edges are removed with the rongeurs in preparation for closure.

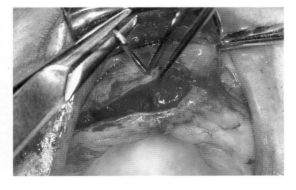

Closure

The first suture replaces the corner of the flap.

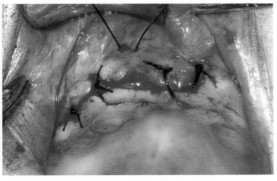

The incision is closed with interrupted sutures but tends to gape where it is unsupported by bone, so a mattress suture is used to reinforce the apposition of the edges.

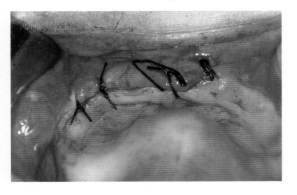

The knot is tied firmly, but not tightly, and the cut ends are left longer than those of the interrupted sutures in order to make it easier to distinguish them at the time of removal.

Follow-up

Healing was uneventful, and the new denture construction was commenced a few weeks later.

10   Cysts

Enucleation of multiple dental cysts

FS, a 62-year-old retired shipyard worker, developed a painful swelling at the front of his mouth, beneath the upper denture. Preliminary radiographic assessment revealed a cyst in the right upper incisor area. The patient was hypertensive and reported penicillin hypersensitivity. The active infection responded to a 5-day course of erythromycin (250 mg, four times daily). Further radiographic assessment showed that there were in total four radiolucent cystic areas, two in the right maxilla and two in the left mandible. It was agreed that the four lesions should be enucleated under local anaesthesia.

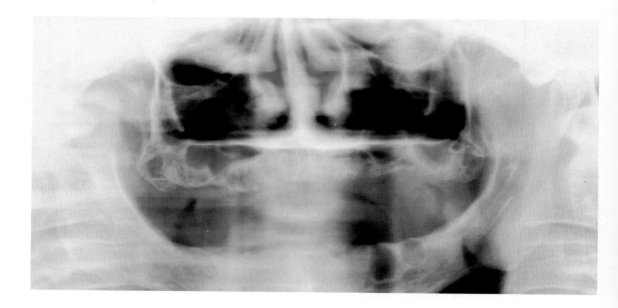

Radiographic assessment

The outline of the cyst in the right upper anterior region can be seen clearly on the orthopantomograph, but the extent of this lesion and the presence of another smaller one in the premolar area are more accurately delineated on the occlusal film. The mandibular lesions are sufficiently well demonstrated by the orthopantomograph. The deepest parts of the bone defects are close to the inferior dental canal.

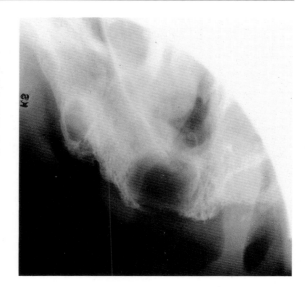

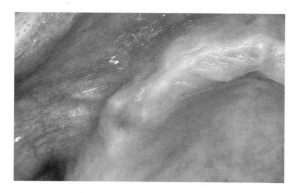

Operation

Operation site: upper cysts

The edentulous ridge is fairly smooth and the mucosa is healthy.

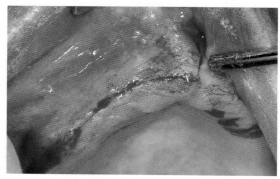

Incision

The incision is made slightly buccal to the crest of the ridge, commencing distally to the position of the distal cyst (estimated with reference to the radiographs) and ending anteriorly, with a short relieving incision just to the left of the midline.

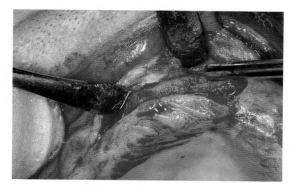

Reflection

The flap is raised buccally, using two Howarth's periosteal elevators.

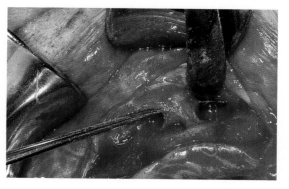

There is a fibrous scar at the site of a previous discharging sinus, which indicates the position of the cyst beneath the bone surface. The subperiosteal tissue plane is opened around the tethered area, and the band of fibrous tissue is freed from the bone surface with a scalpel.

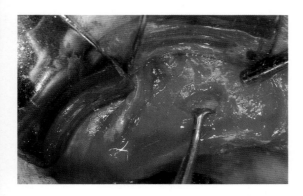

Exposure

The thin bone overlying the cyst is picked away with a Mitchell's trimmer.

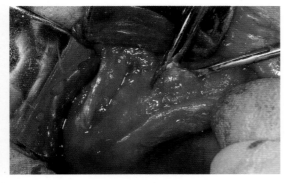

Delivery

The curette is scraped around the smooth cortical wall of the bony cavity, easily freeing the cyst capsule which can then be scooped out in one piece.

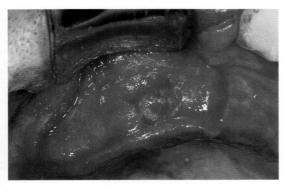

The bony defect can be slightly saucerized by trimming sharp edges, but gross bone removal is unnecessary.

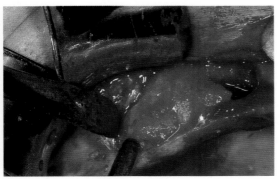

The second cyst was found when the thin covering bone was picked away with the spike end of the Mitchell's trimmer.

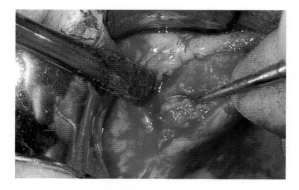

The cyst is delivered in the same way as the first.

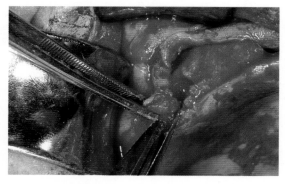

It needs to be cut free from the overlying mucosa with scissors.

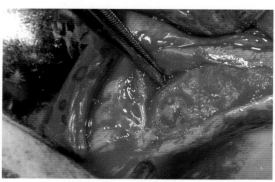

The bony cavity is left to fill with blood clot.

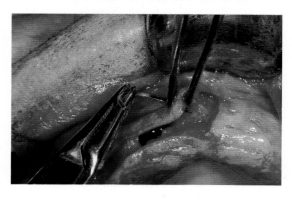

Closure

The first suture replaces the anterior corner of the flap.

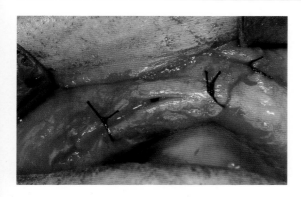

The second suture closes the relieving incision and the third bisects the length of the incision.

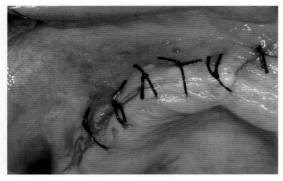

Further sutures close the remaining parts.

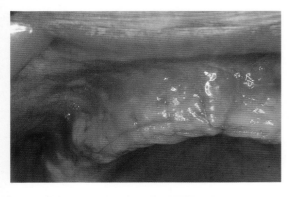

Follow-up

Healing was successful.

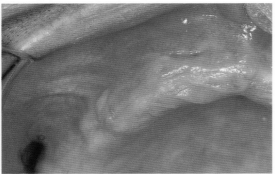

One month later, no trace of the surgery can be seen.

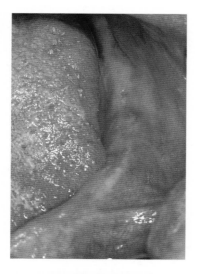

Operation site: lower cysts

The lower ridge is quite bulky, but the extent of attached gingival tissue is limited.

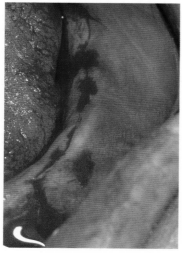

Incision

The incision runs from the retromolar pad forward, to a point well anterior to the estimated position of the anterior cyst.

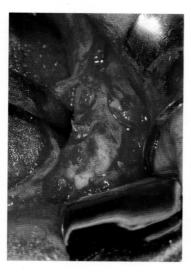

Reflection

The soft tissues are reflected buccally and, to a limited extent, lingually. The position of the cysts is revealed by defects in the bony cortex.

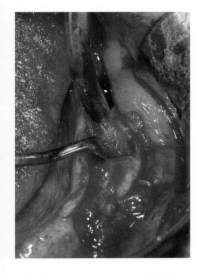

The posterior cyst is curetted out.

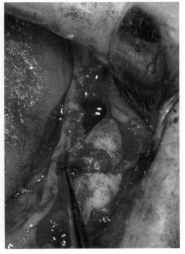

The anterior cyst is freed.

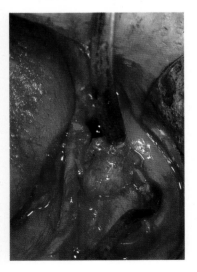

It is drawn from the wound on the sucker tip. Care is required in removing small tissue pieces in this way, since they may disappear into the tubing!

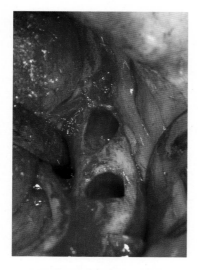

The clean bony cavities are allowed to fill with blood clot.

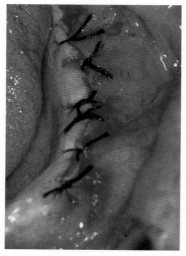

The flap is sutured back in its original position.

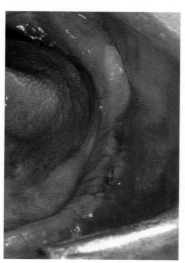

Follow-up

A week after operation, the incision lines have healed well.

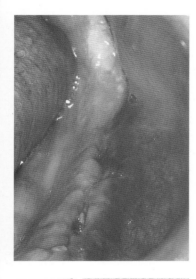

Long-term healing was satisfactory and new dentures were provided.

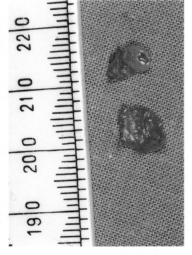

Pathology report

The cysts are shown with a millimetre scale. The specimens were placed in bottles of formal saline and, together with clinical and radiographic details, were sent for histopathological examination.

Maxillary cysts

The cyst from the upper central incisor area was found to be lined by nonkeratinized stratified squamous epithelium, consistent with a residual cyst. The cyst from the premolar area, which had a small root fragment attached to it, showed the features of a periapical cyst.

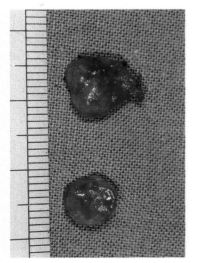

Mandibular cysts

The pathologist remarked that both cysts showed essentially the same appearance, with linings of nonkeratinized stratified squamous epithelium, consistent with residual cysts.

Mucocele

ED, a 26-year-old lawyer, was referred by his general medical practitioner, whose advice he had sought about a painless swelling of his right lower lip. His medical history was clear, but he mentioned that he had noticed 'glands in his neck' which were palpable — especially when he had a cold. A few cervical lymph nodes could be palpated but, in view of his obvious good health, he was simply advised to consult his physician if the problem persisted. The lip lesion was a typical mucocele and the patient was reassured of its harmless nature. He agreed to its removal under local anaesthesia.

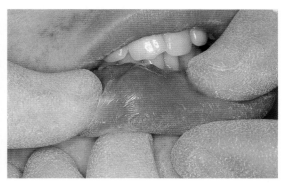

Operation

Operation site

The lesion is visible in the right lower lip. The assistant's fingers hold the lip firmly and, to reduce the blood supply to the area, firm but gentle pressure is applied on either side of the working area.

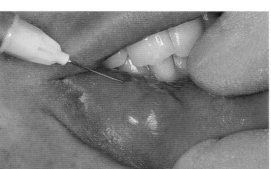

Local anaesthetic infiltration beneath and around the lesion not only anaesthetizes the area, but reduces bleeding by vasoconstriction.

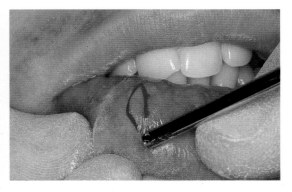

Incision

An elliptical incision is made, through the mucosa only, over the dome of the lesion. This isolates a patch of mucosa overlying the thin friable cyst lining, which is robust enough to be grasped with toothed forceps. Incidentally, the elliptical shape also eases the straight line closure of the mucosal defect.

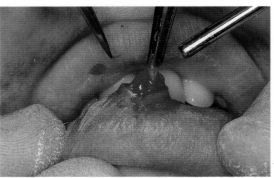

The elliptical patch of mucosa is grasped with toothed forceps and upward traction applied.

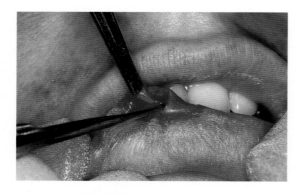

Dissection

Sharp-pointed scissors are inserted, with the blades closed, into the tissues between the cyst and the mucosa.

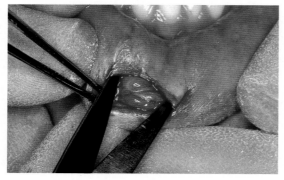

The tissues are blunt-dissected away by opening the blades.

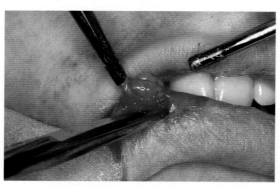

A steady upward traction is maintained, and eventually the cyst is freed.

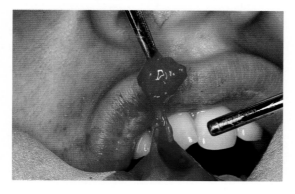

There are usually some berry-like minor salivary glands attached to the base of the lesion, and these are also snipped free with scissors.

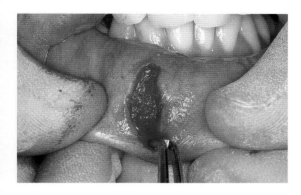

Closure

The underlying connective tissue and muscle can be seen in the base of the wound. Control of bleeding is still being aided by the assistant's finger pressure.

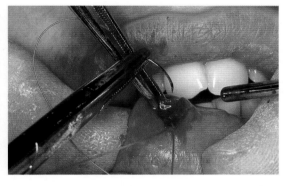

A sheet of connective tissue is grasped in the forceps and sutured to a similar layer, on the other side of the wound, using a 3/0 catgut suture.

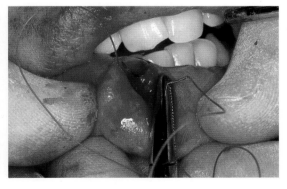

The needle passes from beneath the edge of the sheet of tissue on the first side, and then from above the sheet of tissue on the second side. In this way, when the knot is tied, it retracts deep to the connective tissue layer and is buried in the wound. The ends are cut very short.

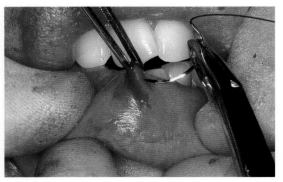

The mucosal layer is closed with black silk sutures, tied in the usual way. The first suture is placed halfway along the incision.

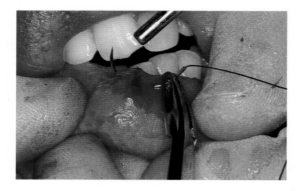

Generous 'bites' of tissue can be taken, as this will assist approximation and eversion, and also prevent post-operative bleeding.

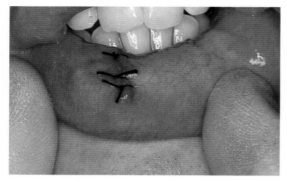

The wound has closed easily with only three sutures.

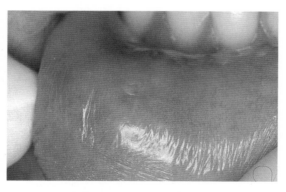

Follow-up

At suture removal, 5 days later, healing is already almost complete.

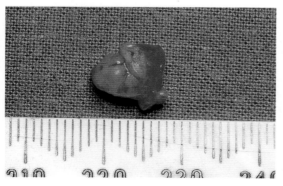

The intact lesion is despatched for histological examination. The lobulated cystic shape is apparent, as are the minor glands attached to the deep pole. When a mucocele bursts during removal – as they often do – here is no choice but to remove, approximately, the right amount of tissue and a few neighbouring minor glands for good measure. Accurate dissection is really only possible if the mucocele remains intact.

Soft tissue biopsy

Biopsy of a tongue papilloma

MJ, a 28-year-old discotheque manager, presented for removal of his impacted lower third molar. He also reported having noticed a small lump on the right side of his tongue which had been present for some weeks. On the basis of the clinical appearance, the patient was reassured as to the benign nature of the lesion, but it was agreed that it should be excised for biopsy. The clinical diagnosis was papilloma.

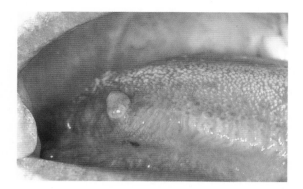

Operation

Operation site

The lesion, which was about 5 mm in diameter, was situated on the right side of the closure of the tongue, just anterior to the foliate papillae.

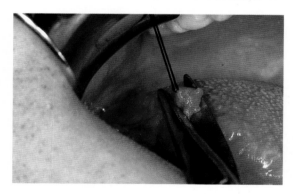

Excision

The lesion was transfixed with a suture.

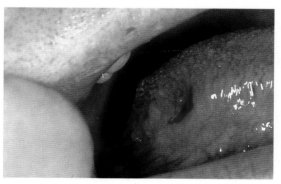

It was elevated and cut free with scissors. The small defect stopped bleeding after a few minutes and did not require a suture. The patient was advised to return a week later to check healing, and to be informed of the outcome of the histopathological examination.

Pathology report

The specimen was found to consist mainly of epithelium, which was hyperplastic and showed the features of a squamous cell papilloma. The pathologist remarked that the possibility of HIV infection should be considered in such lesions found in an unusual intra-oral situation in young males. (There was no other evidence of possible HIV infection and this comment was not divulged directly to the patient.)

Biopsy of hyperplastic nodule

MS, a 45-year-old community organizer, was being examined with a view to the provision of new full dentures to replace those she had worn for many years, when an area of hyperplastic tissue was found in the right mandibular premolar region, lying just buccally to the edentulous ridge. The patient agreed to leave out the lower denture and, after a few weeks, the lesion had considerably reduced in size. A small lump remained, and its excision was advised. Although taking thyroxine therapy, the patient was fit for minor oral surgery under local anaesthesia.

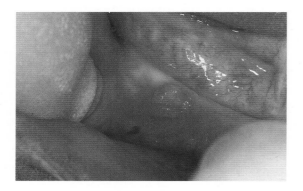

Operation

Operation site

Although now small and shrunken, the lesion retains its original bilobed shape. It lies just at the edge of the attached gingival tissue of the narrow fibrous ridge. The base has been infiltrated with local anaesthetic.

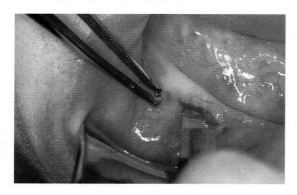

Excision

The most pendulous portion is excised.

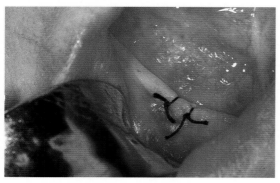

The remaining leaf of tissue is undermined and mobilized.

It is drawn to the other edge of the wound to produce a neat closure, without undue tension across the suture line.

Follow-up

The rearrangement of tissue meant that an insufficient amount of tissue had been excised to form a useful biopsy specimen, but this is acceptable in the case of a lesion so obviously benign. Healing was uneventful and impressions for new dentures were taken a few weeks later.

Excision of palatal fibro-epithelial polyp

JM, a 65-year-old housewife, had been aware since childhood of a small lump in her palate, but had resisted surgery for it. However, she was advised that its presence would complicate the provision of a new denture and she therefore agreed to excision under local anaesthesia. The clinical diagnosis was fibro-epithelial polyp, with pleomorphic salivary adenoma as a possibility.

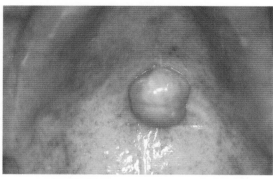

Operation

Operation site

The base of the lesion was infiltrated with local anaesthetic solution.

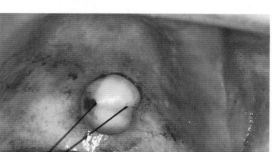

Excision

The lesion is transfixed with a suture, which is used to pull it to each side in turn.

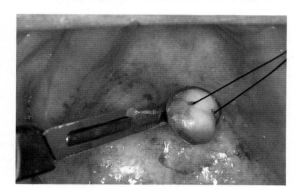

The stalk can be cut free with the scalpel.

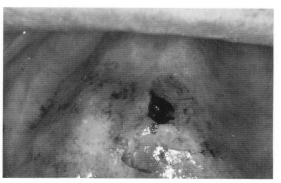

The residual defect is roughly elliptical in shape.

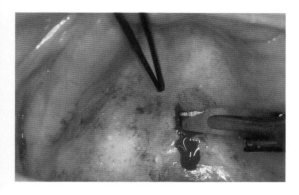

Closure

The edges of the wound are undermined to ease closure.

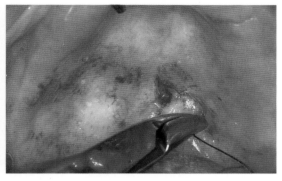

The needle is held end-on in the Gillies' needleholder and a generous bite of tissue taken.

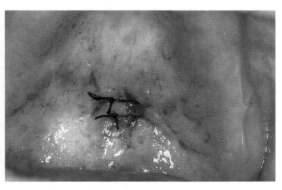

Two sutures suffice to close the wound.

Follow-up

When examined, one week later, the sutures have been shed spontaneously and, despite the inflamed appearance, there were no complaints and healing was satisfactory.

Pathology report

Histological examination showed an area of simple fibrous overgrowth covered by a mildly keratotic epithelium. The features were in keeping with the clinical diagnosis of a fibro-epithelial polyp.

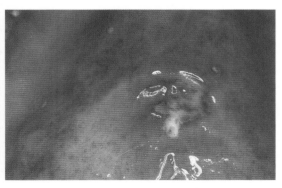

Oro-antral communication and displaced root

CJ, a 36-year-old security man, attended with a complaint of toothache in his upper left second molar. During its extraction, the buccal roots were displaced into the maxillary sinus, but the palatal root was removed successfully. Radiographs confirmed the presence of a displaced root fragment in the sinus, and it was agreed to proceed immediately to remove it under local anaesthesia. The nature of the problem, and its possible consequences, were explained to the patient, who appeared unconcerned.

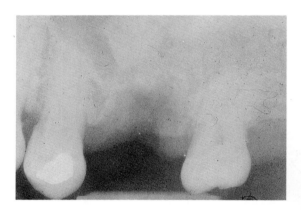

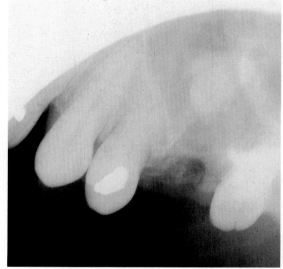

Radiographic assessment

The periapical film shows the displaced double root apparently lying just above the socket, within the sinus cavity. The occlusal film confirms this information and shows the two root canals particularly clearly. As the films have been taken at slightly different angles, there can be no doubt that displacement is minimal and the root should be readily accessible through the socket. The occipito-mental film does not show the displaced root but demonstrates a radiopaque area in the lower part of the left maxillary sinus, which otherwise appears to be healthy and of similar radiolucency to the right side.

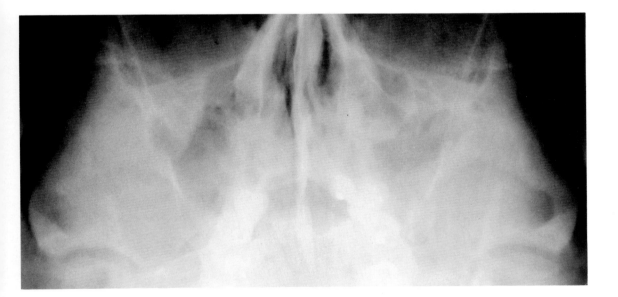

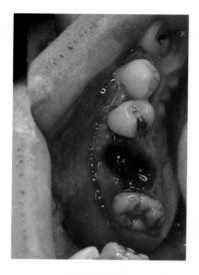

Operation

Operation site

The socket of the upper right second molar is filled with blood clot and the buccal gingival margin is intact.

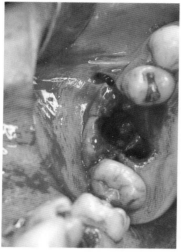

Incision

Two short relieving incisions are made across the gingival margin towards the sulcus.

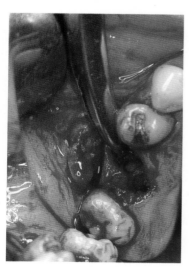

Delivery

A few loose fragments of bone are removed from the socket. Thanks to efficient suction and the precise direction of the operating light, the root can just be seen lying in the sinus, not far removed from its original position.

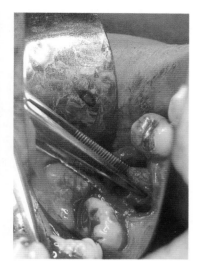

The root can be grasped with fine straight forceps.

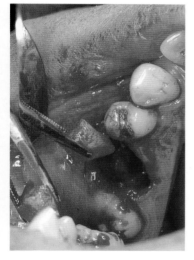

The root is withdrawn.

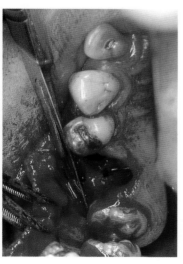

Closure

The periosteal lining of the flap is incised antero-posteriorly to allow it to be drawn across the socket without tension.

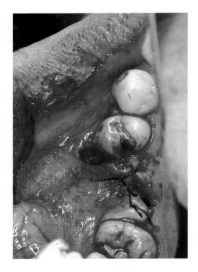

The first two sutures appose the corners of the flap to the palatal socket margin.

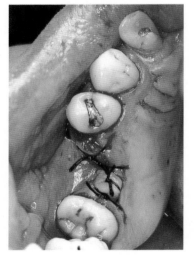

Further sutures repair the buccal relieving incisions and close the central portion of the wound.

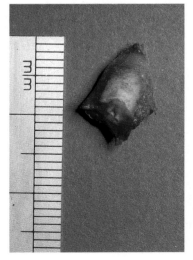

The root with its attached bone fragment is retained and photographed for medico-legal reasons.

Follow-up

The wound healed without difficulty, and there was no residual fistula. The patient accepted that the problem arose through misfortune rather than negligence.

Chronic oro-antral fistula

SM, a 51-year-old school secretary, had a dental clearance, followed by generally satisfactory healing. However, a socket persisted in the upper left molar region, through which she noticed the passage of air when blowing her nose. There was some pain in this region after the extractions, but it gradually settled. When examined in the clinic 6 months later, a fistula could be probed. There was little local inflammation and no discharge. She was generally fit, although occasionally taking lorazepam for anxiety. She agreed to have the fistula closed under local anaesthesia.

Radiographic assessment

A periapical film shows the persistent outline of a molar socket with an impression of discontinuity of the outline of the sinus floor. In cases such as this, periapical films serve mainly to exclude the presence of a retained root.

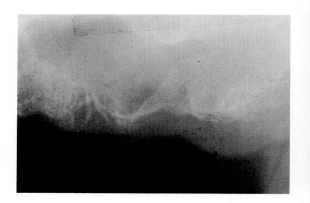

The occipito-mental view shows partial opacity of the left maxillary sinus. This is probably due to swelling of the sinus lining where contamination through the fistula is most frequent. The right sinus is quite clear.

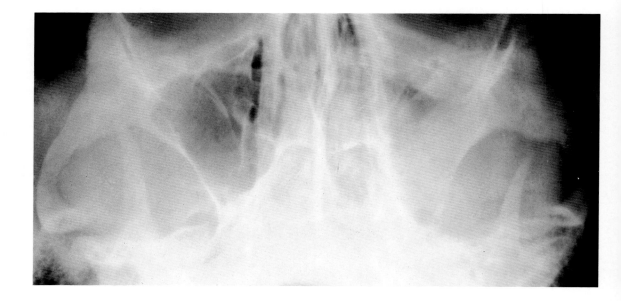

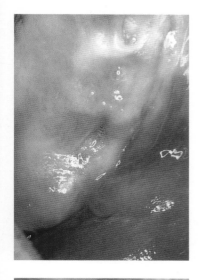

Operation

Operation site

The alveolar mucosa is pale and healthy, and the ridge still demonstrates the outlines of the sockets of the teeth extracted 6 months previously.

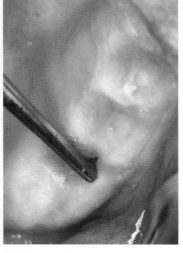

A probe (in this case, the spike end of a Mitchell's trimmer) is used to demonstrate the site of the fistula – at the base of a small depression of the ridge.

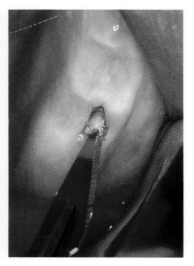

Incision

The epithelialized edge of the fistula is first excised, using a no 11 blade.

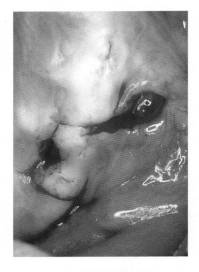

An incision incorporating this defect is made for about 1.5 cm along the crest of the alveolar ridge. From each end a relieving incision is made, starting at a right angle and then diverging into the buccal sulcus, so as to give a broad base for the flap.

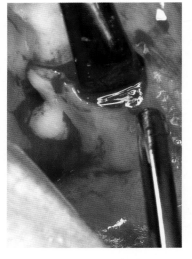

Reflection

A Howarth's periosteal elevator is inserted subperiosteally and used to separate the flap from the bone, starting buccally and working up beneath the attached gingival edge.

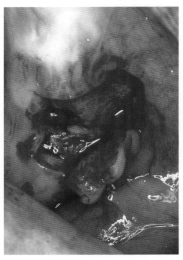

The underlying bony defect can now be seen, partially occluded by inflamed sinus lining.

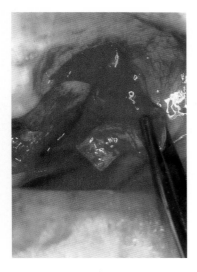

The periosteum is deeply undermined to free the flap.

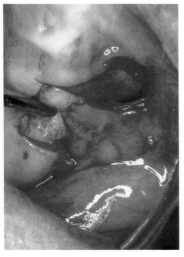

The flap can be replaced across the defect, but broad surface contact can only be obtained at the cost of tension across the wound.

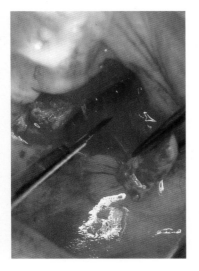

Periosteal incision

The tough inelastic fibrous periosteal layer is incised to relieve the tension.

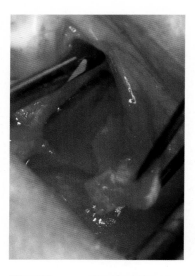

The buccal mucosal layer is extremely elastic and easily extensible. The cut edge of the periosteum can clearly be seen, as can the degree of release already achieved. The anterior edge is finally severed with the scalpel.

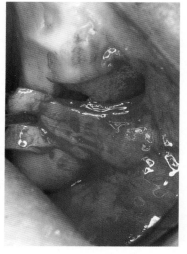

Traction on the flap with the tissue forceps gives a feel for the degree of movement and, when the periosteal incision is completed, the flap can be advanced, without creating tension, across the defect and beyond. Even large defects can be closed readily in this way.

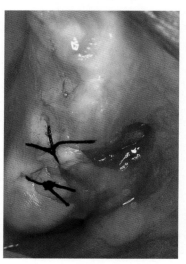

Closure

The first two sutures are placed obliquely across the angles of the incision to anchor the corners of the flap.

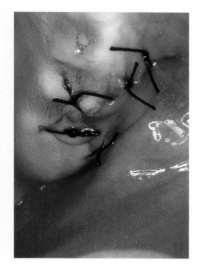

The next three sutures close the anterior and posterior relieving incisions.

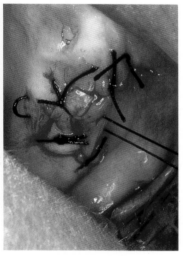

Final broad approximation of the edges is achieved by the insertion of a horizontal mattress suture.

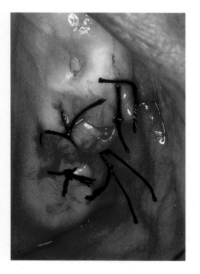

The ends of this suture are cut longer than the others so that they can be identified at the time of removal. The precise number and placement of sutures varies from case to case, but this general order will suit for most.

Follow-up

Sutures were removed 10 days later, and satisfactory healing was achieved.

Appendix A
Instruments

The set of instruments illustrated is, quite simply, the kit that was used for all the operations illustrated in this book. Everyone has his or her own favourites, but this represents a basic selection which has been in use for many years in a busy department. None should be difficult to obtain from reputable dental or instrument suppliers, although the original source varies both in specialty and in nationality. Similar instruments available in the USA are listed where appropiate.

Top row, left to right

- 2 towel clips
- metal aspirating cartridge syringe
- disposable needle
- cartridges of 2% lignocaine with 1/80 000 adrenaline (US: 2% lidocaine with 1/80 000 epinephrine)
- mirror
- probe
- tweezers
- 5 gauze swabs, 10 cm × 10 cm

Second row, left to right

- aspirator tip and matching stilette
- Kilner cheek retractor (US: Minnesota retractor)
- scalpel handle with disposable blade (no 15)
- 2 Howarth's periosteal elevators (Howarth's nasal raspatory; US: Molt no 9 periosteal elevator)
- Mitchell's trimmer (Cumine scaler is similar)
- straight handpiece
- no 6 rose-head bur (steel or tungsten carbide; US: no 6 round bur)
- no 6 tapered fissure bur (tungsten carbide; US: no 701 tapered fissure bur)
- cloth sleeve
- 2 plastic gallipots

Third row, left to right

- Warwick-James' elevators – right, left and straight (US: Miller no 73 and no 74 or Potts elevators)
- 2 Coupland's chisels – medium and small (US: no 301 and no 34S elevators)
- 2 Cryer's elevators – right and left
- upper universal extraction forceps
- rongeurs
- disposable plastic irrigating syringe

Bottom row, left to right

- small mosquito artery forceps
- large straight artery forceps
- Gillies' needleholder
- Mayo needleholder
- Gillies' tissue forceps
- disposable suture, 3/0 silk on 3/8 cutting needle
- small sharp-pointed scissors

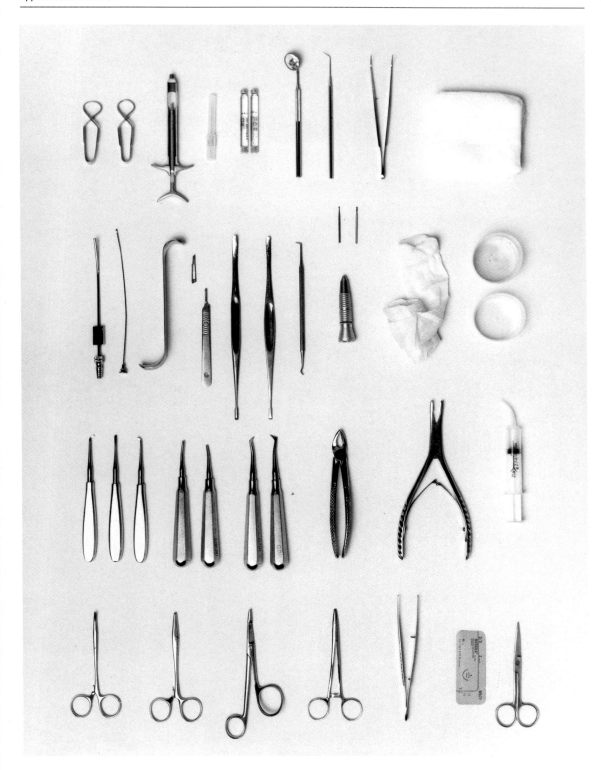

Appendix B
Medicaments and materials

Only a few simple, inexpensive medicaments and materials are required. All are available from a pharmacist if not already in the surgery stock.

- sterile normal saline – for irrigation of wound
- 0.2% chlorhexidine – for preparation of skin and mucosa or postoperative irrigation
- buffered formal saline (in suitable containers) – for pathological specimens
- gauze swabs, 10×10 cm
- periodontal packing material
- cotton wool rolls
- sutures – silk, gut
- 1 cm ribbon gauze
- iodoform paint
- sterile resorbable oxidized cellulose

Appendix C
Sample postoperative advice leaflet

ADVICE TO HELP YOU RECOVER QUICKLY

The operation wound in your mouth requires just as much care as it would anywhere else in your body. It needs to be left alone as far as possible for the first 24 hours so that the initial healing is undisturbed. From that time on, the aim is to keep it clean so as to try to avoid infection.

Pain – should be relieved by simple painkillers like aspirin, paracetamol or ibuprophen.

Swelling – mild swelling is a natural effect of surgery and will go down in a few days.

Stiffness – is caused by a protective spasm of the jaw muscles and will also take a few days to disappear.

Bleeding – should not occur after your return home.

General activity – be sensible and have an early night for once!

Cleaning – clean wounds heal best. Regular tooth brushing (as best you can) and rinsing with warm salty water will speed your recovery.

IF YOU HAVE A PROBLEM OR ARE WORRIED ABOUT YOUR PROGRESS, PLEASE DO TELEPHONE ME FOR ADVICE

Recommended reading

Medical background

Cawson R A, Curson I, Whittington D R, The hazards of dental local anaesthetics, *Br Dent J* (1983) **154**:253–8.

Davidson Sir Stanley, *The Principles and Practice of Medicine*, 15th edn (Churchill Livingstone: Edinburgh 1987).

Scully C, Cawson R A, *Medical Problems in Dentistry*, 2nd edn (Wright: Bristol 1987).

Report of a Working Party of the British Society for Antimicrobial Chemotherapy, The antibiotic prophylaxis of infective endocarditis, *Lancet* **ii(8311):** 1323–6.

Surgical texts

Barnes I E, *Surgical Endodontics* (MTP Press: Lancaster 1984).

Howe G L, *Minor Oral Surgery*, 3rd edn, (Wright: Bristol 1985).

MacGregor A J, *The Impacted Lower Wisdom Tooth* (Oxford University Press: Oxford 1985).

McGowan D A, James J, *The Maxillary Sinus*, (Wright: Bristol, in preparation).

Index

EAST GLAMORGAN GENERAL HOSPITAL
CHURCH VILLAGE, near PONTYPRIDD